THE
THYROID
BOOK

THE
THYROID
BOOK

MARTIN I. SURKS, M.D.

CONSUMER REPORTS BOOKS

A Division of Consumers Union

YONKERS, NEW YORK

Copyright © 1993 by Martin I. Surks
Published by Consumers Union of United States, Inc., Yonkers, New York 10703.

Library of Congress Cataloging-in-Publication Data
Surks, Martin I.
The thyroid book / Martin I. Surks.
p.   cm.
Includes index.
ISBN 0-89043-584-7
1. Thyroid gland—Popular works.   I. Title.
RC655.S84   1993
616.4'4—dc20   93-5245
CIP

Design by Abby Kagan

Third printing, December 1995
This book was printed on recycled paper. ♻
Manufactured in the United States of America

The Thyroid Book is a Consumer Reports Book published by Consumers Union, the nonprofit organization that publishes *Consumer Reports*, the monthly magazine of test reports, product Ratings, and buying guidance. Established in 1936, Consumers Union is chartered under the Not-for-Profit Corporation Law of the State of New York.

The purposes of Consumers Union, as stated in its charter, are to provide consumers with information and counsel on consumer goods and services, to give information on all matters relating to the expenditure of the family income, and to initiate and to cooperate with individual and group efforts seeking to create and maintain decent living standards.

Consumers Union derives its income solely from the sale of *Consumer Reports* and other publications. In addition, expenses of occasional public service efforts may be met, in part, by nonrestrictive, noncommercial contributions, grants, and fees. Consumers Union accepts no advertising or product samples and is not beholden in any way to any commercial interest. Its Ratings and reports are solely for the use of the readers of its publications. Neither the Ratings, nor the reports, nor any Consumers Union publications, including this book, may be used in advertising or for any commercial purpose. Consumers Union will take all steps open to it to prevent such uses of its material, its name, or the name of *Consumer Reports*.

*This book is dedicated to my patients.
Caring for them has always been the most
personally rewarding experience among all
of my professional responsibilities.*

CONTENTS

ACKNOWLEDGMENTS

I wish to thank Roslyn Siegel, Senior Developmental Editor, Consumer Reports Books, for her continuous guidance and encouragement, and the Editors of Consumer Reports Books for their help in preparing the manuscript.

INTRODUCTION

At least 10 million Americans have been diagnosed with thyroid disease, and it is certain that many others suffer from it. Despite the high frequency of thyroid disorders in the population, the public is generally uninformed about the symptoms produced by thyroid dysfunction. Indeed, a majority of Americans probably do not even know where the thyroid gland is located or what it does.

Public awareness regarding thyroid function and disease has increased recently because of the publicity given to the Bush family. Barbara Bush, and later President George Bush, developed an overactive thyroid due to Graves' disease. Detailed information concerning their illness, its diagnosis, and the treatment was presented on the front pages of newspapers around the world, and it led more patients to seek medical attention for various thyroid conditions.

One of my goals in writing this book is to provide easily understood information for the general public about the thyroid and its diseases, in order to enable people to obtain better medical care. My experience as a consultant in endocrinology has shown that although most patients with thyroid disease can be simply diagnosed and their treatment managed successfully, they may not get proper treatment because of their own fears and the fact that some physicians are not current in the diagnosis and management of thyroid diseases. Some patients are advised to have unnecessary and expensive diagnostic tests and surgery; others have unrealistic expectations or excessive fear of the implications of their diagnosis, causing them to change physicians frequently or even to avoid medical care.

This book will inform patients about proper diagnosis and treatment, and can lead to a more productive relationship between patients and their physicians.

1

THE THYROID GLAND: AN OVERVIEW

The thyroid, located in the front of the neck, was first described by Galen, the famous Greek physician (A.D. 130–200) who believed that its role was to facilitate speech by supplying a fluid to lubricate the larynx, or voice box. The actual function of the thyroid, however, was not discovered until the latter half of the nineteenth century, when physicians recognized that surgical removal of the thyroid gland in both animals and human beings resulted in a similar clinical disorder, *myxedema.** It was soon noticed that such symptoms as swelling of the body, sluggishness, low body temperature, and slow pulse, which were found in patients with postsurgical myxedema, could also be seen in patients who still had their thyroid glands. This led to the conclusion that myxedema was caused by an underactive thyroid (hypothyroidism) that could

---

*Definitions of all words in italics can be found in the Glossary.

3

occur either spontaneously or after surgical removal of the thyroid gland. It was then hypothesized that myxedema was caused by the absence of a substance produced by the thyroid gland and secreted into the body.

Within only a few years, thyroid deficiency in patients with myxedema was reversed, first by feeding them whole thyroid glands obtained from animals, then by giving thyroid extracts of dried, powdered glands. Discovering the cause of myxedema and determining how to reverse the disorder was one of the first instances of a successful medical treatment based on careful scientific observation.

THE ENDOCRINE SYSTEM

The thyroid is one of the components of the *endocrine system*, a network of glands that regulates many of the body's most complex and vital functions. Other endocrine glands include the pituitary, the pancreas, the adrenals, the parathyroids, and the gonads (the ovaries and the testes).

All of these glands produce *hormones*—chemical substances with the ability to produce changes in tissues and organs that are distant from the glands themselves. For example, the hormone testosterone is produced in the testicles but influences the growth of facial hair and muscles in men, as well as causing the voice to deepen.

The endocrine glands differ from the many other glands in the body (such as the sweat glands and the salivary glands) because they are *ductless*: They do not contain tubes or ducts that deliver their products. The hormones produced by the endocrine glands are secreted directly into the bloodstream and quickly circulate throughout the body.

LOCATION AND STRUCTURE

Your thyroid gland is closely related to several firm structures in the front of your neck that are relatively easy to find (Figure 1.1). The main structure is the *thyroid cartilage*, which contains your *larynx*, or voice box. (In men, the thyroid cartilage contains the Adam's apple.) Your thyroid cartilage will also be the uppermost bonelike structure in the middle of the front of your neck, and will vibrate when you say "ahhh." Just below your thyroid cartilage is a firm, broad band called the *cricoid cartilage*. Below it are a number of narrower, firm rings that form the front of your *trachea*, or breathing tube. The thyroid gland usually contains two distinct lobes, one on each side of the neck, which are joined across the middle of the neck by a narrow band of thyroid tissue called the *isthmus*. If you remember that your thyroid isthmus crosses the

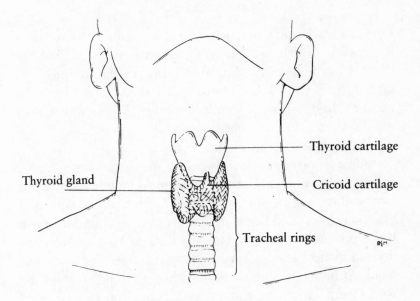

Figure 1.1. Anatomy of the thyroid gland

middle of your neck around the level of the cricoid cartilage, you will know that your thyroid lobes are adjacent to it, located either right on the front of the trachea or at the sides of the trachea. Each thyroid lobe is a little over one inch long, and the lobes are generally quite soft. Because of this soft texture, a doctor may not be able to feel a normal thyroid gland.

FUNCTION

The thyroid gland can be considered to be a chemical manufacturing plant that not only produces and stores thyroid hormones but also delivers them in the correct amount to your body each day.

Iodide Accumulation

One of the thyroid's unique features is its ability to accumulate iodide, which is actually an integral component of the thyroid hormones (see chapter 2). One of the thyroid hormones, *thyroxine* (T_4), contains four iodide atoms, while the other thyroid hormone, *triiodothyronine* (T_3), contains three iodide atoms. Iodide constitutes about 60 percent of the weight of these two hormones.

Iodide is a trace element found in the earth's crust, and it is distributed unevenly around the world. While many areas have sufficient iodide in the ground, in the water supply, and in food products, iodide is in scant supply in other locations. If the production and secretion of thyroid hormones by the thyroid gland varied according to the iodide supply, people would produce too much thyroid hormone in areas of the world with large amounts of iodide and too little thyroid hormone in areas of iodide scarcity. The result would be wild fluctuations in thyroid hormone production and secretion that would be detrimental to the normal day-to-day function of the body's tissues and cells.

However, since your thyroid requires a certain amount of iodide every day, it has developed a remarkable and very efficient mechanism to actually concentrate iodide from the low concentration in your blood. When appropriately stimulated, thyroid cells can even improve the efficiency of the iodide-concentrating (trapping) mechanism when severe iodide deficiency occurs.

Thyroglobulin Production

All cells in the body are capable of manufacturing proteins from smaller building blocks called amino acids, and all cells contain the genes that provide the chemical code for each protein. Although each cell in the body has genetic information about all possible proteins, individual cells produce only a specific set of proteins. *Thyroglobulin* is a protein made only by thyroid cells. Most thyroglobulin is found in your thyroid gland, but some enters the bloodstream, where it is easily measured. The unique production of thyroglobulin in thyroid cells makes measurement of blood serum thyroglobulin a helpful guide in managing some patients with thyroid cancer (see chapter 17).

Thyroglobulin is of critical importance to thyroid cells because it is within this protein that the thyroid hormones are made. After iodide in the body is trapped by thyroid cells, it is introduced chemically into some of the amino acids that are part of the thyroglobulin protein molecule. Several of these amino acids combine to form the thyroid hormone molecules T_4 and T_3. At this point, T_4 and T_3 are actually part of the protein structure of thyroglobulin.

Storage and Secretion

Another unique feature of your thyroid gland is that it stores a large amount of thyroid hormones but secretes just the right amount necessary for normal body function each day. Your thyroid gland is actually composed of innumerable small spheres called *follicles*. The surface of each sphere, or follicle, is composed of a single layer of thyroid cells. The interior of these thyroid follicles is filled with a liquid that contains protein (called *Colloid*). This protein is mainly thyroglobulin made by your thyroid cells, and it contan T_4 and T_3. Normal individuals may have as much as a one-to-three-month supply of thyroid hormones stored in the colloid.

When your thyroid cells are appropriately stimulated, they take microscopic droplets of the colloid back into the cell. The thyroglobulin in these droplets is then broken down into its constituent amino acids, including the thyroid hormones T_4 and T_3. Most of the amino acids that are released from thyroglobulin reenter the blood plasma or are reutilized by thyroid cells for the manufacture of new thyroglobulin molecules. The thyroid hormones T_4 and T_3, however, enter the circulation and are distributed widely throughout the body. The body closely regulates the amount of colloid taken back into thyroid cells and the amount of thyroid hormones secreted into the circulation (see chapter 3).

2

THE THYROID HORMONES

The thyroid hormones thyroxine (T_4) and triiodothyronine (T_3) are called organic chemicals because they are made of carbon, hydrogen, oxygen, and nitrogen atoms, which are similar components to most other constituents of the body (including proteins, fats, and carbohydrates). As noted previously, the thyroid hormones differ from all other hormones because they also contain iodide atoms, which are essential for their biological activity.

HOW THEY ARE PRODUCED

The normal thyroid gland produces mostly T_4, which is secreted into the bloodstream and circulated throughout the body. In various organs such as the liver, kidney, pituitary, and brain, T_4 molecules come into contact with specific proteins called *enzymes* that remove one of the four iodide atoms of T_4, thereby creating a new chemical, the hormone T_3. Thus, T_3 can be produced in two ways: directly in your thyroid gland, as is T_4, or *from* T_4 with the help of enzymes in various organs. Normally, most of the T_3 in the body is made from T_4 with the help of those enzymes and not by the thyroid gland.

HOW THEY ARE REGULATED

The thyroid's production and secretion of T_4 and T_3 are regulated by *thyrotropin*, the thyroid-stimulating hormone (TSH). TSH, which is critically important for the normal, day-to-day functioning of the thyroid gland, is produced by the anterior pituitary gland. This gland, located at the middle of the base of the brain, just behind the eyes, is known as the "master gland" because it regulates the function of the other endocrine glands. After TSH enters the bloodstream, it is widely distributed throughout the body but affects only the thyroid gland. TSH stimulates virtually every function of the thyroid cells, causing them to trap more iodide, to make more thyroglobulin and thyroid hormones, and to secrete more thyroid hormones into the circulation. TSH is the most potent known growth factor for thyroid cells, a fact that is very important in the treatment of patients with thyroid nodules and thyroid cancer (see chapters 16 and 17, respectively).

COMPLEX INTERACTIONS

The pituitary gland itself is influenced by hormones produced by the hypothalamus, a small area at the base of the brain connected to the pituitary by a narrow stalk. The pituitary's production of TSH is controlled by a hypothalamic hormone called *thyrotropin-releasing hormone (TRH)*. TRH causes the immediate release of TSH into the circulation.

The complex hormonal interactions between the hypothalamus, the pituitary, and the thyroid results in the secretion of just the right amount of thyroid hormones for your body's needs each day.

HOW THEY REGULATE TSH LEVELS

An important action of thyroid hormones on the pituitary gland allows the body to maintain relatively constant blood concentrations of these hormones. This process is called *negative-feedback regulation of TSH*, and it operates something like a thermostat (see Figure 2.1).

If concentrations of thyroid hormones should rise above normal levels in the blood, there is a resultant decrease in TSH secretion and, subsequently, a decrease in secretion of

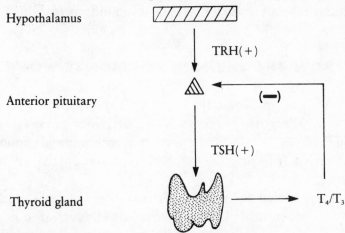

Hypothalamus

TRH(+)

Anterior pituitary

(—)

TSH(+)

Thyroid gland

T_4/T_3

Figure 2.1. Thyroid hormones regulate TSH. TSH stimulates the thyroid gland to produce the thyroid hormones T_4 and T_3, which, in turn, regulate TSH secretion.

thyroid hormones. Eventually, the levels of T_4 and T_3 in our bloodstream return to normal.

By the same token, when the concentrations of thyroid hormones in the blood fall below normal levels, secretion of TSH and the thyroid hormones is increased until T_4 and T_3 are restored to normal levels.

HOW THEY ARE TRANSPORTED

Most of the T_4 and T_3 that circulates throughout your body is tightly bound to proteins in the plasma (the fluid portion of the blood that remains after the red and white blood cells are removed). The proteins that transport the thyroid hormones throughout the body are specific to thyroid hormones because they have within their structures certain shapes and chemical characteristics into which T_4 and T_3 fit like keys in a lock. Most of the T_4 and T_3 in the blood will circulate throughout the body attached to these proteins, leaving only a small amount of each hormone unbound, or *free*.

HOW THE THYROID HORMONES WORK

If you have an overactive or underactive thyroid, you will have a variety of symptoms. Moreover, your physician will find widespread physical effects due to abnormal amounts and activities of the many proteins regulated by thyroid hormones.

After thyroid hormones enter cells, some of the T_4 and T_3 bind to cell proteins known as *thyroid receptors*. (See Figure 2.2.) These in turn interact with the regulatory segments of genes, resulting in an increase or decrease in the concentration of specific messenger RNAs that contain the genetic code for

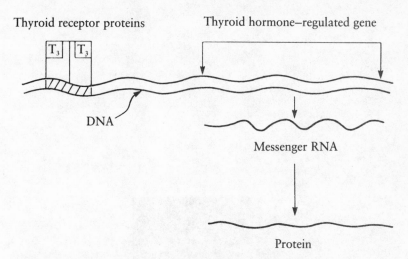

Figure 2.2. Thyroid hormone (T_3) regulates genes and proteins. Thyroid receptor proteins with bound T_3 interact with regulatory regions of specific genes, changing their activation and the concentration of their corresponding messenger RNA and proteins.

individual cellular proteins. Since proteins carry out many of the functions of the body, their regulation by thyroid hormones is crucial for normal cell function. Thyroid diseases associated with increased or decreased serum T_4 and T_3 therefore result in severe cellular dysfunction.

THE EFFECTS OF THYROID HORMONES

Thyroid hormones influence virtually all of the organs in the body. In patients with thyroid disease, the skin, hair, and nails will undergo important physical changes. The muscles are also markedly influenced by fluctuations in thyroid hormones; muscle weakness is a symptom of hyperthyroidism, and cramping occurs in hypothyroidism. In almost all patients with thyroid dysfunction, the effects of thyroid hormones on the brain are apparent. Patients with hyperthyroidism become nervous and irritable, and have short attention spans, whereas patients with hypothyroidism have a dull intellect and blunted emotional reactions. Another prominent feature of patients with thyroid disease is bowel dysfunction: More-frequent bowel movements occur in hyperthyroidism, whereas constipation is characteristic of hypothyroidism.

METABOLISM

Each cell in the body contains several thousand proteins. Some of these proteins provide the superstructure that enables the cell to maintain its size and shape; some help the cell generate chemical energy; and others assist the cell in carrying out its specialized functions. The generation of chemical energy is particularly important because energy is required both to maintain body temperature and to sustain all cellular functions. The two fuels used to produce the chemical energy of the cell are carbohydrates and fats. They are taken up from the blood into all cells and are broken down by a complicated series of chemical reactions, all controlled by proteins called enzymes. The breaking down of glucose and fats requires oxygen and results in the production of chemical energy—the only energy source available to carry out many of the cells' functions. The rate at which food is broken down, oxygen is utilized, and chemical energy is generated is called the *metabolic rate*. That rate is controlled by thyroid hormones.

If your thyroid hormone blood levels are too high (hyperthyroidism), your metabolic rate will be increased, resulting in an increase in the generation of chemical energy and an increase in heat production as well. Because of this excessive heat production, you will feel warm even when others do not, and you will perspire excessively.

If you have an underactive thyroid (hypothyroidism), you will have a decrease both in metabolic rate and in heat production, and you will then feel uncomfortably cold even in warmer temperatures.

THE HEART

The changes in metabolic rate that occur in thyroid disease are paralleled by changes in the function of the heart. An increase in the metabolic rate, induced by hyperthyroidism, requires that your blood circulate more quickly throughout your body so that more oxygen can be delivered to the different organs.

Both the rate and the force of each contraction of the heart are directly influenced by thyroid hormones. If you are hyperthyroid, you will have a fast heart rate even while resting, and contractions will be stronger. As a result, you will experience palpitations, which are sensations of abnormally rapid heartbeat, or you will feel in your chest the thrust of the abnormally strong force of each beat.

Arrhythmias

The excessive stimulation of the heart by thyroid hormones when you are hyperthyroid may result in several serious consequences. You may develop abnormal changes in the rhythmic pattern of your heartbeat, known as *arrhythmias*. The most commonly encountered arrhythmia in hyperthyroidism is *paroxysmal atrial fibrillation*, a condition in which the heart is beating so rapidly and irregularly that its ability to fill up with blood and then pump it out to the body is impaired. If the heart rate becomes too rapid, the flow of blood out of the heart may actually begin to decrease.

In atrial fibrillation, blood clots may form in the heart, break loose, and enter the bloodstream. A stroke may eventually result if the clot obstructs an artery that supplies the brain, and significant damage may occur in other organs if their arteries become blocked by blood clots that originate in the fibrillating heart.

Insufficient Blood Flow

Another serious consequence of the heart's pumping faster and harder than normal is that it requires more oxygen and blood. The heart receives its own supply of blood, which is delivered through the coronary arteries. If you have significant narrowing of the coronary arteries due to arteriosclerosis, and you are also hyperthyroid, this narrowing of the coronary blood vessels may prevent the increase in blood flow and oxygen needed by your heart. Insufficient blood flow to your heart under these circumstances may result in chest pain (angina pectoris) or, occasionally, even a heart attack (myocardial infarction).

HUMAN GROWTH AND DEVELOPMENT

Abnormalities of growth and development do not generally concern adult patients with thyroid disease, but they are of paramount importance in children. Normal blood levels of thyroid hormone are necessary for the pituitary gland to produce normal amounts of growth hormone.

It is therefore not surprising that a child's growth is impaired whenever he or she develops hypothyroidism prior to puberty—even if the anterior pituitary is quite normal. If not treated, such children have abnormally short stature. When hypothyroidism has been present from birth and goes untreated, a type of dwarfism develops called *cretinism* (see chapter 19).

THYROID DISEASE AND MEDICATIONS

One of the consequences of an increased or decreased metabolic rate is that your body will eliminate certain medications more rapidly or more slowly than before. When you are treated with medication, the concentration of the drug in your body depends on the amount you take, how frequently you take it, and the rate at which the body eliminates it. Drugs are eliminated either by the destructive action of enzymes, by excretion of the drug into the urine or feces, or by a combination of these processes. Since thyroid hormones regulate the overall rate of metabolism, they also regulate the elimination rate of many drugs. Therefore, if you are taking various medications when you develop thyroid disease, your physician will have to determine whether the dosage of your medication needs adjustment to compensate for changes in drug elimination rates. Always inform your physician if you are taking medication prescribed by another doctor.

THE DOCTOR'S EXAMINATION

Many thyroid disorders can readily be managed by your internist or family physician, but some should be managed by an endocrinologist. For example, the diagnosis and treatment of primary hypothyroidism is usually straightforward and can be handled by any well-trained family physician or internist. In contrast, the evaluation of thyroid nodules or goiter and the management of thyroid cancer should probably be done by an endocrinologist who has substantial experience with these disorders. Other thyroid problems, such as hyperthyroidism resulting from Graves' disease, can be managed by your internist in consultation with an endocrinologist when changes in treatment plan, particularly radioactive iodide therapy, are contemplated.

CHOOSING A PHYSICIAN

Although these suggestions are generally valid, the experience of your personal physician in treating thyroid disease is always an important consideration in determining whether you should be treated by your own doctor or by a consulting endocrinologist. You, as the patient, should therefore play an active role in ascertaining the qualifications of your physician.

Under ideal circumstances, you will have had a long experience with your physician, resulting in a relationship based on mutual respect and trust. You will expect your doctor to tell you whether he or she feels competent to treat your disorder, or whether you require the knowledge and experience of a specialist.

Unfortunately, many patients do not have a long-standing relationship with any one physician. In this situation, you must seek assurance that the doctor you consult has sufficient experience to treat your thyroid disorder.

The quality of medical education varies widely, both in medical school and at the postgraduate level, and many training programs stress patient care in a hospital setting. Since thyroid disorders do not often call for hospitalization, many doctors, even if trained in good schools and postgraduate programs, have little experience in diagnosing and caring for patients with thyroid disorders. Therefore, you or your advocates must directly ask your doctor about his or her experience with your disorder; ask for a referral to an endocrinologist if your doctor's experience with your condition is limited.

If you have no personal physician and you think you may have a thyroid disorder, you should probably first visit an internist for a complete medical evaluation, including appropriate blood tests. The internist may then refer you to an endocrinologist. One guide to the quality of the doctor that you select is board certification, evidence that the physician has completed an approved training program and then has taken a rigorous examination that tests his or her competence. Passing that examination certifies that a physician has appropriate training, a base of knowledge, and suitable personal qualities to practice that specialty.

You can ask your doctor directly about board certification or you can review the doctor's qualifications in various directories available in almost all medical libraries and in most good general libraries. See the appendix for the names of directories that list the qualifications of all physicians in the United States. The appendix also provides a list of professional and lay organizations that will help you find a qualified physician.

When You Visit the Doctor

Your medical history. When you visit your physician because of a particular complaint, describe the timing, frequency, intensity, and duration of your problem as completely as possible. Your physician should be able to elicit more information by asking you specific questions. Since the susceptibility for developing some thyroid diseases runs in families, questions concerning the presence of thyroid disease in other family members is an essential part of establishing your medical history.

It is a good idea to make a written list of your symptoms and any questions you may have, then bring that list with you when you see your doctor. It's also often helpful if a family member accompanies you when the doctor takes your medical history. That person may be able to prod your memory or provide more details about your illness, helping your doctor to get a clear idea of all your symptoms.

The establishment of your medical history is a critical part of the continuing relationship between you and your doctor. By listening carefully to what you have to say and by asking the appropriate questions, your doctor will have a solid foundation for making a correct diagnosis.

The thyroid examination. Examination of your thyroid gland is a central component of the physical examination for thyroid disease. The physical findings not only establish the presence of disease but also provide important insights into its causes.

Your doctor will look carefully at the area of your neck that contains the thyroid gland. You will usually be sitting up with your chin raised and your neck muscles relaxed. You will probably then be asked to swallow. If you feel your own thyroid cartilage or trachea as you swallow (see Figure 1.1), you will notice that each will go up and down as part of the swallowing mechanism. Since your thyroid gland is attached to your trachea, it will also go up and down when you swallow. The swallowing maneuver is an important part of the examination. A normal thyroid will usually not be visible when you swallow. If your thyroid is enlarged or contains lumps called *nodules*, such abnormalities are often first noted during this careful inspection of your thyroid area.

Your doctor may feel your thyroid gland while standing behind you or standing face-to-face with you. Some physicians will do both. In either case, you should be able to feel your doctor's fingers along the sides of your trachea at the level of your cricoid cartilage and inside your neck muscles. When the tips of the physician's fingers are at the sides of your trachea, you will be asked to swallow. Some physicians will feel both of your thyroid lobes simultaneously. Others may push your trachea toward one side of your neck while grasping the opposite lobe between the thumb and fingers.

A combination of these maneuvers should determine

whether your thyroid is normal or enlarged, whether the texture and consistency of your gland are normal, and whether or not nodules or masses are present. A normal thyroid may be sufficiently soft in consistency that your doctor cannot feel it. If your doctor does not ask you to swallow when his or her fingers are appropriately placed along the sides of your trachea, it could result in failure to detect significant abnormalities.

After feeling your thyroid, your doctor may also listen to the gland with the stethoscope. You will be instructed to hold your breath while the doctor listens for whooshing sounds known as *bruits*, which would indicate a large increase in blood flow to the gland.

General physical examination. Since thyroid disease can affect all systems of the body, your doctor will carry out a general examination to determine whether you have signs of thyroid dysfunction. Your height, weight, pulse rate, and blood pressure should be recorded. Skin temperature, texture, and moisture will be noted. Examination of the head, eyes, ears, nose, and throat may provide important clues about the state of your thyroid. The eyes, in particular, will be evaluated for signs of thyroid orbitopathy (see chapter 7). Fingernails will be examined, and the outstretched fingers will be evaluated for shaking or tremors. Examination of your heart, lungs, and abdomen, as well as your neurological system, including your reflexes (which are determined by tapping over your tendons with a reflex hammer), also provide important information for your physician.

There are specific signs that your doctor knows are associated with either an overactive thyroid (see chapter 6) or an underactive thyroid (see chapter 11). The constellation of these signs, together with your medical history and your doctor's findings on examination of the thyroid, will help him or her decide the nature of your thyroid condition. All of this information will then allow your physician to order the most appropriate laboratory tests to confirm the findings obtained from your history and physical examination. This logical sequence will lead to an accurate diagnosis and effective treatment of your condition.

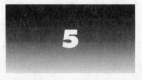

DIAGNOSTIC TESTS

A variety of tests are available for your doctor to determine the precise nature of your thyroid problem. The doctor's selection of the appropriate tests to diagnose your condition will be based on the results of history and physical examination, the specificity of the tests themselves, and their cost. Measurements of thyroid hormones and TSH are the mainstay for determining whether or not you have thyroid dysfunction, and they have generally replaced the more expensive and cumbersome tests that use radioactive iodide.

MEASUREMENT OF T₄

When there is suspicion that you have either an overactive or underactive thyroid, your physician will probably request measurement of thyroid hormone concentrations in your blood, since abnormal concentrations may be signs of a thyroid disorder. It is usually not necessary to measure both T_4 and T_3 to determine the state of thyroid function, because in most instances the blood levels of these hormones rise or fall together in different thyroid diseases. Since most of the hormone secreted by your thyroid gland is T_4, it is logical that the concentration of T_4 in your blood will reflect the function of the thyroid more closely than the serum concentration of T_3, only some of which is secreted by the thyroid.

Your physician will therefore order serum T_4 measurement as the first test of your thyroid function. T_4 measurements almost always provide your doctor with information needed to determine general thyroid function. Concentrations of serum T_4 that are above the normal range are usually associated with an overactive thyroid condition, whereas decreased serum T_4 concentrations usually signify an underactive thyroid.

FREE T_4 MEASUREMENTS

Measurement of serum T_4 includes all the T_4 in your blood—both the T_4 that is bound to serum-binding proteins and the very small amount that is not bound, or free. There are some circumstances when your physician will request a free T_4 determination rather than a serum T_4 determination to assess your thyroid function.

This should be done whenever the physician has reason to believe that the amount of the circulating proteins that transport the thyroid hormones throughout your body has either increased or decreased. When there are more binding proteins in your blood, there are also more thyroid hormones bound to them, and the serum T_4 will be increased. If you do not have thyroid disease, your free T_4 should remain normal even when levels of the binding proteins and total T_4 are raised. Therefore, the free T_4 becomes the best test to measure your thyroid function when the serum-binding proteins are changed. This more refined test is more expensive than the serum T_4 determination.

TABLE 5.1

Causes of Raised Serum-Binding Proteins

Estrogens	Liver Disease	Hereditary
Pregnancy	Acute hepatitis	
Oral Contraceptive Medications	Chronic hepatitis	
Postmenopausal Estrogen Treatment		

SERUM TSH MEASUREMENTS IN THYROID DISEASE

Understanding the negative-feedback regulation of TSH secretion by thyroid hormones from the pituitary gland (see chapter 2) allows doctors to predict changes in pituitary TSH secretion and serum TSH concentration that occur in several common thyroid disorders. A decrease in serum TSH would be anticipated if you have an overactive thyroid producing increased serum T_4 and T_3 blood levels. Conversely, if you have a thyroid disease that results in less than normal secretion of thyroid hormones and subnormal serum T_4 and T_3 concentrations, your serum TSH concentration should be significantly increased.

These changes in serum TSH, predicted from the negative-feedback regulation of TSH, do in fact occur in both hyperthyroidism and hypothyroidism resulting from thyroid disease. Therefore, measurement of serum TSH is an important test to help diagnose thyroid dysfunction. Serum TSH measurements are also important in determining the correct dosage of thyroid hormone, given in pill form, for patients who are receiving the hormone for the treatment of hypothyroidism and thyroid cancer (see chapters 13 and 17).

MEASURING OTHER PITUITARY HORMONES

Both the anterior pituitary and the hypothalamus produce other hormones in addition to TSH. Therefore, hypothalamic and pituitary diseases (such as tumors or growths) can influence the secretion of one or more hormones, producing complex endocrine disorders that require measurement of several endocrine gland functions. A deficiency in the secretion of hypothalamic TRH will produce a decrease in secretion of pituitary TSH, resulting in decreased stimulation of the thyroid (underactive thyroid, or hypothyroidism).

If laboratory results suggest pituitary or hypothalamic disease, your physician will measure other pituitary hormones and carry out imaging procedures (such as CT scans or MRI's) of the pituitary-hypothalamic area to help determine the cause of your endocrine problem (see chapter 12).

THYROID IMAGING TESTS

Other diagnostic tests can be used to produce images of the thyroid and its surrounding structures. These include the thyroid ultrasound or sonogram (see chapter 15); computerized axial tomography (sometimes called CT scan); or magnetic resonance imaging (MRI scan). These tests should not be ordered for evaluation of thyroid dysfunction. They can be helpful for the assessment of thyroid nodules (lumps) that are either benign or malignant (see chapters 15, 16, and 17).

TESTS TO CONFIRM HYPERTHYROIDISM

The most direct and inexpensive way for the doctor to confirm his or her clinical impression of hyperthyroidism is to order measurement of your serum T_4 in conjunction with serum TSH. When your thyroid gland is overactive, it will overproduce thyroid hormones and cause an increase in your serum T_4 concentration above the normal range—more than 12 micrograms per deciliter (>12.0 µg/dl).

If there is reason because of pregnancy, use of oral contraceptives, or postmenopausal estrogen replacement therapy to suspect that your serum thyroid-binding proteins are abnormally increased, your doctor will request measurement of your free T_4, instead of serum T_4, which will be increased to above the normal range.

When a test of free T_4 is ordered, it is not necessary to order a test of serum T_4 because no additional helpful information will be provided. Because increased concentrations of thyroid hormones cause a decrease in TSH secretion by the anterior pituitary, patients with hyperthyroidism almost always show a decrease in serum TSH concentration to less than 0.1 micro International Unit per milliliter (<0.1 µU/ml). The combined findings of a raised serum level of T_4 or free T_4 and decreased serum TSH confirm the diagnosis of hyperthyroidism.

UNNECESSARY TESTS

The following laboratory tests are not required in order to confirm hyperthyroidism:

1.   It is not necessary to measure both serum T_4 and serum T_3 to evaluate overactive thyroid function. If the serum T_4 concentration is increased, the serum T_3 will also be increased

in about 95 percent of patients in the United States with an overactive thyroid. Only occasionally will hyperthyroid patients have normal serum T_4 or free T_4, because their thyroid glands are secreting mainly T_3. A serum T_3 determination is warranted only in those patients. Finding an increase in serum T_3 concentration is not necessary to establish the diagnosis in most hyperthyroid patients who have an increase in serum T_4. Routine ordering of serum T_3 measurements is unnecessary because the test provides redundant information and adds significantly to medical costs.

2.   The radioactive iodide uptake and scan and the thyroid ultrasound evaluation are widely used tests to evaluate thyroid disease. Neither test should be used simply to establish whether or not hyperthyroidism is present; that is more accurately and less expensively accomplished by blood measurements. The radioactive iodide uptake and scan can be useful in establishing the cause of the hyperthyroidism and also in treatment (see chapters 8, 10, and 14).

Do not hesitate to ask your physician why a radioactive iodide uptake or thyroid ultrasound test has been ordered on the first visit, before blood tests confirm the presence of hyperthyroidism. Radioactive iodide uptakes, radioactive iodide scans, and thyroid ultrasound examinations are costly. Since measurements of thyroid hormones in blood taken at your doctor's office will be returned within several days, patients can save money and time by waiting for results of the blood tests.

THE RADIOACTIVE IODIDE UPTAKE TEST

Since the trapping of iodide is an important feature of thyroid cells, measurements of the ability of your thyroid to trap iodide can provide useful information concerning your thyroid function. Small and safe amounts of radioactive iodide can be administered by mouth, either in capsule or liquid form, and the radioactive iodide that accumulates in your thyroid gland is determined by means of a machine that measures radioactive iodide either four hours or 24 hours later. The test can be standardized for either time interval.

Results are then expressed as the percentage of the radioactive iodide administered that is taken up by your thyroid. Patients with an underactive thyroid may have decreased values, and patients with an overactive thyroid may have raised values, indicating that their thyroids are accumulating smaller or greater amounts of iodide than people without thyroid disease.

Radioactive iodide tests were once the most important ways to evaluate thyroid function. During the last 20 years, however, blood measurements of the thyroid hormones T_4 and T_3 and the thyroid-stimulating hormone (TSH), discussed in chapter 2, have become so precise and relatively inexpensive that they have replaced the more cumbersome, expensive, and less exact radioactive iodide tests for the diagnosis and management of thyroid dysfunction. However, radioactive iodide tests are important in the evaluation of goiter (see chapter 15), thyroid nodules (chapter 16), and thyroid cancer (see chapter 17); and to determine the cause of hyperthyroidism.

TESTS TO CONFIRM HYPOTHYROIDISM

When your doctor suspects that an underactive thyroid, or hypothyroidism, is the cause of your complaints, the diagnosis can be simply and inexpensively confirmed by ordering a measurement of your serum T_4 or free T_4 as well as TSH.

The vast majority of patients with hypothyroidism have a

diseased or damaged thyroid gland that is unable to maintain adequate production of thyroid hormones. Such patients will have a decrease in serum T_4 concentration to less than 5 μg/dl and a raised serum concentration of TSH to more than 5 μU/ml (see chapter 11). These two laboratory findings alone are sufficient proof that thyroid hormone deficiency exists and that it is caused by disease or damage to the thyroid gland.

Hypothyroidism is infrequently due to an abnormality in hypothalamic or pituitary function that results in decreased secretion of TSH and inadequate stimulation of an otherwise normal thyroid gland. Laboratory confirmation of hypothyroidism in such cases is obtained by finding a decrease in serum T_4 to below the lower limits of the normal range (less than 5 μg/dl) and either a normal or decreased concentration of serum TSH.

UNNECESSARY TESTS

Neither the thyroid radioactive iodide uptake test nor thyroid ultrasound are necessary to confirm the presence of hypothyroidism. A decrease in thyroidal radioactive iodide uptake is not specific to hypothyroidism because there is considerable overlap between the test results of hypothyroid patients and those of normal individuals. Thyroid ultrasound provides visualization of the thyroid but does not measure thyroid function.

6

THE OVERACTIVE THYROID: HYPERTHYROIDISM

Betty D., a 30-year-old working mother of two boys ages seven and nine, had been in good health until the death of her father eleven months earlier. Her low spirits gradually improved after a month or two but were replaced by feelings of apprehension and anxiety that had become progressively worse during the last several months. She also reported that her "fuse had become short," so that her emotional reactions to ordinary day-to-day events were excessive. Considerable friction had developed between her and her husband and children, who saw that she was extremely irritable.

When she initially consulted her family physician, she was told that she was "physically just fine" but was suffering from a severe grief reaction. Her doctor prescribed a tranquilizer, but it did not significantly relieve her symptoms. During the last several months, she had experienced waves of heat and perspiration and a rapid heartbeat, which she attributed to anxiety attacks. The previous week she was frightened by a very rapid heartbeat that persisted for about an hour and had left her weak and somewhat breathless. Her physician found her heart rhythm to be normal but rapid, and her electrocardiogram showed no abnormalities. The examination showed that she had lost seven pounds in five weeks despite the fact that she believed her eating patterns were unchanged. It was also noted that her hands were hot and trembling and that her thyroid gland was enlarged. Her physician's clinical impression of an overactive thyroid (hyperthyroidism) was confirmed by blood tests, and Betty was referred to an endocrinologist (a physician specializing in diseases of the endocrine glands).

Betty's story is similar to that of many patients with hyperthyroidism. Marked mood swings, anxiety, feeling hot all the time, excessive perspiration, palpitations of the heart, and weight loss are some of the most common complaints of hyperthyroid patients. Yet because these may be symptoms of other diseases or emotional problems, they are often misdiagnosed.

Further questioning revealed that Betty's muscle strength had decreased, her bowel movements now occurred after each meal instead of once a day, and she had noticed shaking in her hands, particularly when she held a cup of coffee. Thus, Betty's illness affected the functioning of her brain, skin, heart, muscles, bowels, and nerves. Taken all together, it was clear that her symptoms suggest thyroid disease.

SYMPTOMS

The widespread symptoms of hyperthyroidism are the result of all the tissues in the body being exposed to increased blood levels of the thyroid hormones T_4 and T_3 (see chapter 3).

1. *Heat Intolerance* When you are hyperthyroid, you usually feel hot all the time, wear less clothing than others in the same environment, and experience intermittent flushing. Heat intolerance and the inability to stand warm environments are common complaints because of the excessive heat production that accompanies an increase in metabolic rate (see chapter 3). An increase in perspiration during the day or the night that would be inappropriate for healthy individuals also occurs.

2. *Skin and Nails* You may notice that your skin has gradually developed a fine, silky smooth texture, with areas of increased or decreased pigmentation.

The rate of nail growth in some hyperthyroid patients may increase, and the nails may become soft and easily torn. The nails of normal individuals separate from the nail beds in a smooth semicircular line that is near to and parallel to the tips of the fingers. When you have been hyperthyroid for many months or years, the line of separation between your nails and the nail beds becomes irregular, making it difficult to keep the nails clean.

3. *Hair* If you have hyperthyroidism, one of the first things you notice is that your hair has become softer and finer and does not take a set or permanent wave as well as it did before. Hair loss may follow, and you may become quite alarmed at the excessive amounts of hair you find on your pillow, on your clothing, on the shower floor, and on your hairbrush. Although hair loss may be confined to specific areas of your head (alopecia areata), widespread thinning is more common. Hair loss may be so extensive that you may consult a dermatologist even before you seek help from your family physician.

The hair loss in hyperthyroidism is temporary; it will stop soon after your thyroid problem is controlled. Complete recovery is the rule.

4. *Gastrointestinal Changes* Almost all patients with hyperthyroidism experience some change in gastrointestinal function, most commonly an increase in the frequency of bowel movements. If you previously moved your bowels once a day, you may now have two or more bowel movements daily, and if you were frequently constipated before you developed hyperthyroidism, you now may have daily bowel movements.

5. *Weight Loss* You will generally lose weight as a result of hyperthyroidism, even though you are not dieting or significantly increasing your physical activity. In fact, weight loss often occurs even though food intake is increased, making hyperthyroid patients the envy of most people who are struggling to maintain or lose weight.

Research on the use of thyroid hormones or related agents for weight reduction has shown that thyroid hormones are not a safe way to facilitate weight loss. Significant weight loss will occur only with an overdose of thyroid hormones, and serious complications of hyperthyroidism could result.

6. *Neurological Symptoms* While the increase in energy that is characteristic of hyperthyroidism might seem to be beneficial, and you "can get so much more done," these changes are offset by a decrease in your ability to concentrate and a feeling of fatigue. If you are hyperthyroid, you may feel that you are "wired" or that "your motor is always running," yet at the same time you experience fatigue and exhaustion. Your pattern of sleep is often disturbed, with frequent waking during the night. You may feel that your adrenaline is still flowing and that you cannot achieve a relaxed state for restful sleep. You may have great difficulty maintaining sufficient focus and concentration to complete your work or studies. You may be jumpy and find it nearly impossible to remain in the same place for any period of time; you are always on the move. Even when sitting, movement of your arms and legs and changes of position in the chair may be frequent. Distortion in your normal speech pattern may result in more rapid speech and impatient responses to questions—without your being aware of the change.

7. *Emotional Response* You may experience some profound exaggeration in your emotional reactions and may be perceived as irritable by family members and coworkers. You will overreact to the little events of everyday life that previously did not disturb you, and the result can be strained relationships at home and in the workplace.

The exaggerated emotional reactions of hyperthyroidism may also be found in various psychiatric illnesses—in mood disorders, for example—so these symptoms alone do not indicate hyperthyroidism. An overactive thyroid will be suspected only when your emotional reactions are evaluated along with other symptoms of hyperthyroidism, especially those produced by the abnormal function of other organs.

8. *Cardiovascular Irregularities* At times of emotional and physical stress, everyone experiences a sudden pounding of the heart in the chest or neck, but it disappears when the stressful event is over. This is part of your normal response to stress and is caused by the increased secretion of the hormone adrenaline (epinephrine) by the adrenal glands. When you are hyperthyroid, you experience similar pounding of the heart, or palpitations, because thyroid hormones directly affect how rapidly and forcefully the heart beats and because the increased metabolic rate in hyperthyroidism requires the heart to pump a larger amount of blood (see chapter 3). Unlike healthy individuals, hyperthyroid patients experience their rapid heartbeat and palpitations during periods of mild stress and even in the absence of it. Some patients report that

their heart rate never seems to slow down, even when they are resting.

When you are hyperthyroid, you may experience all gradations of cardiac symptoms—from a heightened awareness of a rapid, strong heartbeat to palpitations that last for seconds at rest or throughout periods of physical exertion. You may also have persistent palpitations due to abnormal heart rhythms, called arrhythmias (see chapter 3), which are associated with pounding of the heart in your neck and shortness of breath.

Atrial fibrillation, a common abnormality in heart rhythm, occurs in 10 to 15 percent of hyperthyroid patients and results in an irregular as well as rapid heartbeat. Patients with atrial fibrillation are aware of short pauses in their heartbeat followed by a burst of rapid beats, with no overall regular pattern. This abnormal heart rhythm may be episodic (paroxysmal), in which each episode lasts for seconds or several minutes, or it may be continuous. In either case, the experience is generally so striking and frightening that most patients will immediately consult a physician.

Atrial fibrillation is a dangerous arrhythmia of the heart because it may be associated either with heart failure or with the formation of blood clots within the heart. When dislodged, these clots can enter the bloodstream and cause a stroke or damage to other organs.

9. *Muscular Weakness* Muscle weakness, particularly in the muscles around your hips and shoulders, leads to a number of complaints in many hyperthyroid patients. You may experience difficulty in climbing stairs. Your thigh muscles may burn or feel weak or soft, causing you to climb stairs slowly and rest often. When the muscle weakness is severe, you may be unable to rise from a sitting position without the

help of your hands and arms, or be unable to get out of the bathtub without assistance.

When your shoulder muscles are affected, you may not be able to brush your own hair or do physical activities that require maintaining your arms above the level of your head for any period of time.

Although muscle weakness is common and causes some disability in many patients, it is not generally severe enough for patients to seek medical attention.

10. *Menstruation*   If you are a woman of childbearing age when you develop hyperthyroidism, you will generally experience a significant decrease in the duration of your menstrual period. With mild hyperthyroidism, your menstrual flow may decrease from three or four days to one or two, and the amount of the flow on each day may be less than normal. When hyperthyroidism is more severe and present for a long period of time, your menstrual flow may decrease to only one or two days in duration, or it may stop altogether.

Some women who are unaware of their hyperthyroidism and experience one or two days of menses, irritability, heart palpitations, and excessive perspiration may believe that they are pregnant. If pregnancy does occur when you are hyperthyroid, you will be at increased risk for a miscarriage (see chapter 18).

Group of Symptoms

If you suffer from the constellation of symptoms just described, it is probably worth having a consultation with your primary care physician to discuss the possibility of thyroid disease. Graves' disease, as well as other common causes of hyperthyroidism, are discussed in the following chapters.

7

GRAVES' DISEASE

Graves' disease, the most common cause of hyperthyroidism, was first described by Sir Robert Graves as a clinical syndrome in the early nineteenth century, when he published case reports of several patients with enlarged thyroid glands, bulging eyes, and symptoms and signs that are now recognized as hyperthyroidism (see chapter 4). Although we have learned a great deal about Graves' disease in the last one hundred years, there is still much about the disease we do not know. We know the effects and the causes of this hyperthyroidism, but we have not determined how the disease process begins or how to prevent it. Fortunately, we have learned to treat it effectively.

AUTOIMMUNITY: THE CAUSE OF HYPERTHYROIDISM IN GRAVES' DISEASE

Most patients with hyperthyroidism due to Graves' disease have enlarged thyroid glands that, on microscopic examination, seem to result from enlargement of all the thyroid cells. Since all of the cells seem to be in a stimulated state, it is likely that the thyroid gland is being affected by excessive concentrations of either a normal or abnormal stimulator.

The discovery of the essential role of thyrotropin (TSH) in regulating thyroid function (see chapter 2) led many researchers to believe that excessive TSH secretion by the pituitary gland might be the cause of hyperthyroidism in Graves' disease. This idea was studied very simply by measuring the concentration of TSH in serum from hyperthyroid patients with Graves' disease (this test became available in the late 1960s). The very sensitive measurements of TSH that are now available have shown that serum TSH concentrations are undetectable in hyperthyroid patients with Graves' disease, thus eliminating TSH, the natural stimulator of thyroid function, as the cause of Graves' hyperthyroidism.

In the 1940s and 1950s, when the possibility of excessive TSH was under study, the sensitive TSH measurements we have today were not available, and many researchers tried to measure TSH by its stimulating activity in different biological systems. In 1956, researchers in Australia discovered a new thyroid-stimulating agent present in the serum of patients with Graves' disease, the thyroid-stimulating antibody, TSAb. This finding suggested that Graves' disease might be a disease of autoimmunity, due to a malfunction of the immune system. (See Figure 7.1.)

Antibodies are proteins the body produces when it is attacked by bacteria, viruses, or other foreign substances. Antibodies bind to the offending organisms, making it easier for other body proteins or the white blood cells to kill them. Many specialized proteins and white blood cells join together to form this defense system, called the immune system, which recognizes the foreign nature of an infecting organism and directs the production of antibodies against it. The immune system also recognizes that the body's tissues and proteins are not foreign invaders and prevents the formation of antibodies directed against them.

The generation of antibodies that stimulate the thyroid gland in Graves' disease therefore represents a breakdown of the normal immune process—the development of autoimmunity. (See Figure 7.1.)

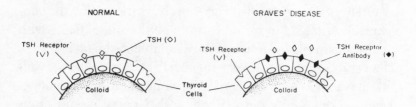

Figure 7.1. Cause of hyperthyroidism in Graves' disease

A. *Normal thyroid:* TSH binds to its receptor proteins on the surface of the cell and stimulates the thyroid gland to produce and secrete thyroid hormones. The thyroid system remains in balance because thyroid hormones, secreted into the bloodstream, decrease TSH secretion.
B. *Graves' disease:* TSH receptors are continuously stimulated by TSH receptor antibodies in an unregulated manner, resulting in overstimulation of the thyroid cells and overproduction of thyroid hormones.

Since antibodies are often generated in response to infection, bacterial agents have been investigated as a cause. No such links have been established, which leads to the conclusion that Graves' disease does not begin with an infection. If you have Graves' disease, you cannot transmit it directly to anyone else.

Graves' disease is not the only autoimmune disease that is recognized; there are many others, including the closely related and common Hashimoto's thyroiditis, which leads to an underactive thyroid (see chapter 12); rheumatoid arthritis; systemic lupus erythematosus; pernicious anemia; and Type I diabetes mellitus.

All patients with hyperthyroidism due to Graves' disease have circulating antibodies that are directed against the TSH receptor protein (Figure 7.1). Since the thyroid cell cannot distinguish whether the TSH receptor protein is interacting with the natural stimulator, TSH, or with an abnormal protein such as thyroid-stimulating antibody (TSAb), it is stimulated in either case to overproduce and oversecrete thyroid hormones. Antibodies, once generated, are slowly removed from the body, so TSH receptors in Graves' disease are continually occupied by TSAb, and the thyroid gland will continually overproduce thyroid hormones.

AUTOIMMUNITY IN GRAVES' ORBITOPATHY

The thyroid-stimulating antibodies that cause hyperthyroidism are probably not responsible for the eye disease that occurs in patients with Graves' disease. In fact, you can have severe hyperthyroidism and no eye disease at all, or have severe eye disease when your thyroid function is normal or only slightly increased. It is uncertain at this time if the eye disorder is really a component of Graves' disease or a very closely related, but distinct, autoimmune disorder.

HEREDITY AND GRAVES' DISEASE

Even though you cannot directly transmit Graves' disease to your loved ones, they will have a higher probability of getting the disease or the closely related Hashimoto's thyroiditis (see chapter 12). This is because the susceptibility of the immune system to malfunction that results in hyperthyroidism is often inherited. If one identical twin develops Graves' disease, for example, the other twin has a fifty-fifty chance of also getting the disease.

It is also true that the chances of developing Graves' disease are about five to ten times greater in women than in men, a pattern that occurs in many autoimmune diseases. The reason for the high susceptibility to autoimmune disease in women has not been discovered. It may be because some genes that are important in regulation of the immune system occur on the X chromosome, which is present only in women. Another theory is that female sex hormones play an important modulating role in the immune system.

Because you have Graves' disease does not necessarily mean that your children, particularly your daughters, will also get it; they will, however, be at a much higher risk for thyroid disease than children from families whose members have no history of thyroid disease.

SMOKING AND GRAVES' DISEASE

Several investigations have shown that patients with Graves' orbitopathy are much more likely to be smokers, raising the possibility that smoking may facilitate the autoimmune reaction that results in Graves' disease and orbitopathy. Although there is no current proof that smoking causes Graves' disease, this possibility may be added to the already long list of medical reasons to stop smoking.

SYMPTOMS

Thyroid Gland Enlargement

The typical patient with Graves' disease has all the symptoms of hyperthyroidism (see chapter 4)—an enlarged thyroid gland, plus specific changes in the eyes.

An enlarged thyroid gland may be the first indication of Graves' disease, appearing before you are aware of any symptoms associated with hyperthyroidism. You may first notice that your neck appears enlarged or feels different to the touch. Often, someone else will be the first to point out the enlargement in the front of your neck. The enlarged gland will not be tender when you touch it or when your doctor feels it during examination.

The thyroid enlargement in Graves' disease may be modest, approximately two times the normal size or even only slightly greater than normal. With such a small degree of enlargement, you may not experience any discomfort, although some patients say that they feel something unusual is there.

If your thyroid gland is very enlarged—about three or four times its normal size—and firm, you may feel a fullness or a slight-to-moderate pressure in the front of your neck. This will be true particularly when you turn your head to the side or when you swallow.

Thyroid gland enlargement in Graves' disease does not usually cause any difficulty in swallowing liquids or solids (dysphagia). If you do experience such difficulty, see your doctor because dysphagia can result from an obstruction or constriction of the esophagus caused by cancer of the throat, esophagus, or thyroid (see chapter 17).

When you have Graves' disease, your doctor will be able to feel your enlarged thyroid and with a stethoscope often will hear a noise over your thyroid called a bruit. This is caused by the greatly increased blood flow through your thyroid gland. If your thyroid is enlarged to a small degree or if the texture of the gland is particularly soft, the enlargement may not be detected by your physician—and occasionally not even by an endocrinologist.

Orbitopathy

It is generally known that eye problems can develop when you have thyroid disease. Doctors will use various terms when referring to the changes in the eye due to Graves' disease: *ophthalmopathy, exophthalmos,* or *thyroid orbitopathy.*

Ophthalmopathy simply means that there is some type of eye disorder; exophthalmos implies that the eye is being pushed forward; and orbitopathy indicates that the problem lies within the orbit, the bony socket of the skull that contains the eyeball, the muscles that move the eye, the arteries and veins that carry blood to and from the eye, and the optic nerve, which transmits visual signals from the eye to the brain. Orbitopathy seems the most appropriate term to use in connection with Graves' disease, since the disorder can affect all of the structures in the orbit.

Orbitopathy occurs in one-half of patients with Graves' disease; its severity varies from barely detectable eye involvement with minimal symptoms to a severe disorder that can compromise vision.

When your thyroid gland swells, even to several times its normal size, few symptoms develop from its increased size because the enlarged thyroid simply stretches the skin and muscles that surround it. Only a slight feeling of pressure in the front of the neck is felt by most patients. However, because the orbit of the skull that contains the eye and the eye muscles is bony, any increase in pressure caused by enlargement of the eye muscles can only be dissipated in one direction—forward—pushing out on the eyeball. The increase in pressure behind the eye interferes with the drainage of blood from the eyeball and eye muscles through the veins of the orbit; this causes congestion and swelling of the eyelids and an increase in pressure within the eyeball itself.

Severe Orbitopathy

Fortunately, only a small percentage of patients with Graves' disease have orbitopathy severe enough to threaten their vision. The six small muscles that move the eye are particularly affected by an inflammation (not an infection) that causes the muscles to swell and become the target of cells from the bloodstream. These cells usually accumulate in chronic inflammations. The muscles that move the eye are normally like thin, flat ribbons, but in severe thyroid ophthalmopathy they may swell to five to ten times their normal size. (See Figure 7.2.)

The size of the enlarged eye muscles may increase to such an extent that the pressure behind the eye causes malfunction

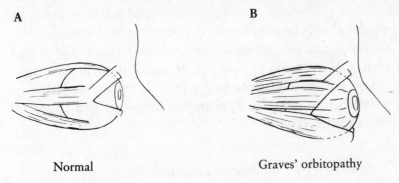

A

B

Normal

Graves' orbitopathy

Figure 7.2. Orbitopathy
A. Normal eye.
B. Eye of a patient with Graves' orbitopathy. The muscles that move the eye are swollen, pushing the eye forward. The eyeball is also congested and irritated.

of the optic nerve. Color vision becomes impaired first; eventually visual acuity will decrease as well. Patients with 20/20 vision may experience a decrease in their vision to 20/40 or 20/80 or worse, if the disease continues its course.

When severely affected eye muscles become weak, movement of both eyes may become uncoordinated, resulting in double vision, or *diplopia*. If you have severe orbitopathy, you may look at a single object and see two objects—one next to the other or one above the other. You will not know which image represents the actual position of the object and which image is false. Double vision clearly complicates all activities of daily living, whether at home or in the workplace. Driving a car becomes impossible.

If you have significant protrusion of your eyes, you and your doctor should be certain that your eyes close sufficiently when you are sleeping to cover the cornea, the transparent surface at the front of your eye, which is very sensitive to drying. An uncovered cornea that is allowed to dry at night can develop painful ulcerations, making you susceptible to infections that can compromise your vision.

When you have Graves' disease and orbitopathy, you should always be alert for the development of changes in color vision and acuity of vision or of double vision and a new feeling of irritation in your eye. If any of these problems develop, you should immediately consult with your physician or endocrinologist for appropriate diagnosis and treatment (see chapter 9).

Pain or Discomfort

If you have thyroid orbitopathy, you may feel varying degrees of aching pain in your eyeball and a dry, irritated feeling in your eye. Some patients feel as if there is sand in their eyes, while others are hypersensitive to bright light, particularly sunlight. Wind, or even the gentle airflow felt by walking, may be irritating, causing the eye to tear incessantly. When you look into the mirror, you may see that you have developed a stare because of the raising of your upper eyelids. This upper-eyelid contraction can occur in patients with any kind of hyperthyroidism. In Graves' disease, additionally, the eye may be pushed forward by the increase in volume and pressure of the contents of the orbit behind the eye. Your eyes may appear red, reflecting congestion, and there may be swelling of tissues that cover the eye (the conjunctiva) as well as the upper and lower eyelids.

Double Vision

When you are examined by your internist or endocrinologist, you will be asked to focus on an object, such as the doctor's finger or a pocket light, that is moved up, to each side, and down again to determine whether you see two objects instead of one. Such double vision would indicate weakness in one or more of the muscles that move your eyes. Your doctor will also examine the surface of your eyes to determine whether there are scrapes or abrasions on your cornea and also to determine how far your eyes are protruding from your skull by making a measurement with a device called an *exophthalmometer*. The doctor may be able to see the white of your eye between the pupil and the upper lid when you move your eyes downward. This is known as a lid lag (see chapter 9), because of the lifting of the upper eyelids due to increased adrenalinelike activity that occurs in hyperthyroidism. Changes in sharpness of your vision and color vision will also be recorded.

DIAGNOSIS

If you are hyperthyroid and have some degree of orbitopathy in both eyes, it is almost certain that it is due to Graves' disease. If both of your eyes are pushed forward, a condition called *proptosis*, and you do not seem to have symptoms and signs of an overactive thyroid, it is still possible that you have mild, clinically inapparent hyperthyroidism caused by Graves' disease.

The severity of the orbitopathy is not necessarily related to the severity of the hyperthyroidism. Many patients with severe hyperthyroidism have no detectable orbitopathy, and some patients with very mild hyperthyroidism may have severe eye disease. It is also possible that the bulging of your eyes is not due to Graves' disease. A stare because of protrusion of both of your eyes, without swelling, redness, blurring of your vision, or eye pain can occur if you are severely nearsighted, have lost a significant amount of weight, have certain liver disorders, have become obese, or have been treated with large doses of cortisonelike drugs.

TESTS

If you go to an internist or endocrinologist because you notice only protruding eyes and a stare, and your doctor does not detect any symptoms or signs that suggest hyperthyroidism, he or she will probably order blood tests to determine whether you have clinically inapparent hyperthyroidism (see chapters 7 and 8). If hyperthyroidism is not detected by blood tests, your doctor will evaluate the size of your eye muscles using an imaging technique such as ultrasonography, computerized tomography (CT scan), or magnetic resonance imaging (MRI). Your eye muscles will be visibly enlarged if Graves' disease is the cause of the proptosis.

All of these procedures will detect very enlarged eye muscles. However, the CT and MRI scans are more sensitive for detecting minimal eye muscle enlargement, and they provide much more detail than ultrasonography.

Your doctor will choose the most appropriate test for you depending on the condition of your eyes, the availability of machines to do the test, and cost factors. Ultrasonography generally costs between $100 and $200, CT scans between $300 and $500, and MRI scans between $700 and $1,000. If ultrasonography of the orbits determines that the eye muscles in both of your eyes are enlarged, the diagnosis of Graves' disease will be established without the need for more expensive procedures.

Although Graves' disease is the most common cause of hyperthyroidism, particularly when it runs in the family, it is not the only cause. There is a 50 percent chance that the telltale Graves' orbitopathy will not be present with the other symptoms discussed in chapter 6. The doctor examining you may find only hyperthyroidism and an enlarged thyroid. The diagnosis of Graves' disease can, however, easily be decided by determining that the 24-hour uptake of radioactive iodide by your thyroid has increased (see chapter 8). The radioactive iodide uptake test is expensive and should be used only if your doctor is uncertain whether you have Graves' disease or hyperthyroidism due to another cause (see chapters 10 and 14).

Although the cause of the hyperthyroidism in Graves' disease is a circulating thyroid-stimulating antibody, measurements of TSAb are not routinely done to determine the diagnosis. The tests are difficult and expensive in comparison to the relatively simple measurements of thyroid hormones and TSH.

Once a definitive diagnosis of Graves' disease has been made, effective treatment can begin.

8

TREATMENT OF GRAVES' HYPERTHYROIDISM

Although we cannot eliminate TSAb, the specific cause of Graves' hyperthyroidism, in the same way that we can kill the bacteria that cause pneumonia, we can still effectively treat the illness by controlling the excessive production of thyroid hormones.

This was once accomplished by surgical removal of most of the thyroid gland. The approach today is either to destroy the thyroid tissue with radioactive iodide (I^{131}) or to prescribe antithyroid drugs that actually interfere with the formation of thyroid hormones. Although neither of these treatments specifically corrects the immunological abnormality that underlies production of TSAb, both remedies will relieve symptoms of hyperthyroidism and restore your thyroid function to normal. Each approach to treating hyperthyroidism has side effects and long-term implications that should be considered along with the benefits of treatment before a decision is made for a specific therapy.

PATIENT PARTICIPATION

Since there are some risks as well as benefits associated with both radioactive iodide and antithyroid drug therapy, and differences in the long-term consequences from both treatments, you should be an active participant in choosing one over the other.

If you have hyperthyroidism, you should ask your doctor about the benefits, risks, and outcome (both in the short term and the long term) of these treatments and not feel rushed into making a decision. Treatment with radioactive iodide is destructive to your thyroid and therefore irreversible, whereas antithyroid drug therapy does not damage your thyroid gland. If you have trouble making the final decision, you should probably be treated initially with antithyroid drugs, which will relieve your symptoms. Drug therapy can always be discontinued and radioactive iodide administered at a later date.

SHOULD YOU BE TREATED?

When your hyperthyroidism is severe and your symptoms significantly interfere with daily activities, there is little question that your disease should be treated. If, however, you are referred to an endocrinologist for treatment and you have few, if any, symptoms suggesting hyperthyroidism, you may well question the need for treatment. A careful history and physical examination may reveal subtle symptoms and findings that are associated with hyperthyroidism. If so, you probably should be treated. If the symptoms or physical characteristics of the condition are not detected, you and your doctor may decide to monitor your hyperthyroidism without specific treatment.

You should be evaluated by your doctor every one or two months initially, both by examination and by measurement of serum thyroid hormones and TSH. Treatment should be started when symptoms or physical characteristics develop or if serum thyroid hormone concentrations begin to rise. In some patients, serum TSH will remain very low even when serum T_4 and T_3 are in the normal range and symptoms or signs of hyperthyroidism are not evident. A recommendation for treatment is controversial in such patients (see chapter 10).

NATURAL REMISSION

In the early decades of the twentieth century, when no specific treatments were available for Graves' disease, studies suggested that over an interval of three to five years, the disease might actually disappear in one-third of all patients. The studies also suggested that the disease would remain relatively constant in its severity in another one-third of patients, while the remaining one-third would face serious disability and even death. Untreated patients who died from the disease usually became emaciated and suffered from abnormal heart rhythms, heart failure, profound muscle weakness, and the consequences of embolization, such as strokes. These potentially serious consequences of hyperthyroidism caused by Graves' disease make it imperative to identify and treat patients with symptoms as soon as possible.

The disappearance of hyperthyroidism without specific

treatment (spontaneous remission) in some patients is an important consideration for selecting the best approach for therapy. If you and your doctor knew at the outset that your hyperthyroidism would never go into spontaneous remission, you might be more likely to select destructive therapy with radioactive iodide. However, if you were sure that your hyperthyroidism would resolve spontaneously—say, within 6 to 12 months—you would more strongly consider controlling the hyperthyroidism temporarily with antithyroid drugs and wait for the remission.

Most autoimmune diseases vary in severity from time to time, and Graves' disease is no exception. While the majority of patients experience constant or increasing severity of their hyperthyroidism, 20 to 40 percent of patients may have only intermittent hyperthyroidism. Remission is more likely if your hyperthyroid symptoms are relatively mild, if your thyroid gland is not greatly enlarged (less than two times the normal size), if the duration of your hyperthyroidism has been relatively short (such as several months), and if your disease followed a severe emotional crisis (for example, a death in your family or loss of your job). If your doctor determines that you have several of these characteristics in common, he or she may be more likely to prescribe treatment with an antithyroid drug rather than to suggest the destruction of your thyroid with radioactive iodide.

ANTITHYROID DRUGS

How They Work in the Thyroid

Two medications—propylthiouracil, or PTU, and methimazole (Tapazole)—are approved for control of hyperthyroidism in the United States. A third member of this group of drugs, carbimazole, is widely used in Europe and Asia. All of these drugs interfere with the formation of thyroid hormones because they interact with an important thyroid enzyme, a protein called *thyroid peroxidase*.

In normal individuals, iodide that is taken up from the blood by the thyroid cells is then incorporated into thyroglobulin, a protein important in the production of thyroid hormone (see chapter 1). Normal activity of thyroid peroxidase is critical for this step in hormone formation. By interfering with thyroid peroxidase, antithyroid drugs decrease thyroid hormone production. At the appropriate dosage, each of the antithyroid drugs is equally effective in decreasing the activity of thyroid peroxidase and, therefore, formation of thyroid hormones.

Many patients have the misconception that they will begin to feel better as soon as they start taking antithyroid drugs. Unfortunately, this is not the case. It is true that antithyroid drugs used in the appropriate dosage will stop production of new thyroid hormone molecules almost immediately, but your thyroid gland usually has a very large reserve of thyroid hormone that was produced before treatment with antithyroid drugs was started (see chapter 1).

The storage capacity for thyroid hormones may be large enough to maintain normal thyroid function for one to three months without forming any new thyroid hormone molecules. Until all the stored thyroid hormones become depleted, the rapid release of the stored thyroid hormones into the blood will maintain the hyperthyroid state. Several weeks to several months of continuous treatment are therefore required before your thyroid hormone reserves are depleted to the point where thyroid hormones in blood and tissues decrease and significant clinical improvement occurs.

Other Effects

PTU exerts a unique effect outside of the thyroid gland, and this results in a decrease in the production of T_3. In contrast to T_4, much of the body's T_3 is made not in the thyroid gland but in the liver and other organs, using T_4 made in the thyroid. This action is facilitated by a protein enzyme, T_4 deiodinase (see chapter 2). PTU, but not methimazole, interferes with the activity of the deiodinase enzyme so that serum T_3 formation is decreased more rapidly during PTU treatment than during treatment with methimazole. Even though this effect of PTU is significant, the length of time before you are restored to normal thyroid function is usually still longer with PTU than with methimazole.

How They Are Prescribed

PTU is available in 50-milligram (mg) tablets, whereas methimazole can be prescribed either in 5- or 10-mg tablets. The initial dosage of antithyroid drugs, sufficient to block almost all new thyroid hormone production, should be 300 to 400 mg of PTU per day or 30 to 40 mg of methimazole per day. Since methimazole is removed from the body much more slowly than PTU, the full daily dosage of methimazole can be taken at one time. PTU is usually prescribed in divided doses: 100 mg or two tablets every eight hours, or three tablets twice per day, for example. Both drugs are completely absorbed from the gastrointestinal tract and can be taken either when your stomach is empty or after you have eaten. Neither is irritating to your stomach or bowels.

Like other medications, it is important that you take antithyroid drugs as prescribed. Lapses in therapy will allow the formation of thyroid hormone at a high rate, increase serum thyroid hormone concentrations, and delay relief of your hyperthyroidism.

Since once-a-day therapy is more easily remembered than several doses per day, methimazole may be best for you if you are occasionally forgetful. Medication containers with compartments for each day of the week are available in most pharmacies, and they may also help you to keep up with your doses. When each of the compartments is filled with the appropriate number of tablets for each day, a glance at the compartment will indicate whether or not you have taken the correct daily dose of your medication. If you do not remember whether you have taken the day's dosage, assume that you have not and take the appropriate dosage at that time. Ingesting a few extra tablets of PTU or methimazole from time to time will not hurt you and will help ensure continuous inhibition of thyroid hormone production, thereby shortening the time it takes to normalize your thyroid function.

Initial Management of Treatment

Dosage adjustment.   Your doctor's strategy for antithyroid drug treatment is to prescribe a dosage that inhibits most of your thyroid hormone formation until your hyperthyroidism is relieved. He or she then decreases the amount of the drug to a maintenance dosage, which is the minimal amount of medication necessary to maintain a normal production of thyroid hormone.

A normal thyroid state, known as *euthyroidism*, generally occurs after four to eight weeks of treatment with methimazole and after 6 to 12 weeks of treatment with PTU. If the dosage of antithyroid drug is maintained at a level that blocks most thyroid hormone production, you will first become euthyroid and then hypothyroid. Therefore, it is important for you to see your doctor every three to six weeks for examination and measurement of serum T_4 and TSH concentrations. The physician can gradually decrease the dosage of antithyroid drugs as you become euthyroid, until a dose is established that maintains you in the euthyroid state.

Maintenance dosage. A maintenance dosage of PTU is generally in the range of 50–150 mg per day; that of methimazole is usually 5–15 mg per day. While on a maintenance dose of antithyroid drugs, you should be evaluated by your doctor every three or four months and eventually at six-month intervals. Your doctor's evaluation will consist of a brief, focused history and physical examination that will be relevant to symptoms and signs of both hyperthyroidism and hypothyroidism, as well as to the side effects of antithyroid drugs (see below). Laboratory tests should include measurement of serum T_4 or free T_4 and TSH, occasional measurement of your white blood cell count, and several tests of liver function. Measurement of the thyroidal uptake of radioactive iodide, thyroid ultrasonograms, X rays, CT scans, or MRI scans is not necessary.

Improvement of symptoms. During the first few months of treatment, you should notice gradual improvement in all symptoms of hyperthyroidism. Your rapid heart rate will slow to normal, your palpitations will disappear, your feelings of warmth and excessive perspiration will improve, your appetite will decrease, your bowel function will normalize, your muscles will become stronger, and you will probably gain some weight. You will likely feel less nervous. In particular, the tremors of your hands and body will disappear and your skin temperature will become normal.

Weight gain. Most patients are gratified with the improvement of their hyperthyroid condition. Nevertheless, since we live in such a weight-conscious society, many are dissatisfied with the weight gain that usually accompanies restoration of the normal (euthyroid) state.

When you are hyperthyroid, your metabolic rate is increased and your body's requirement for different nutrients is much greater than normal (see chapter 3). As your metabolic rate returns to normal during treatment of hyperthyroidism, you will require smaller amounts of nutrients.

Eating patterns are largely based on habit, and you were used to eating large amounts of food without gaining weight when you had hyperthyroidism. This habit may be difficult to change. If you do not want to gain too much weight when your hyperthyroidism is relieved, you should gradually decrease your food intake as your thyroid function becomes normal. After normal thyroid function has been restored and you are taking a maintenance dose of antithyroid drugs for several months, your new eating pattern will likely be established, and your weight should stabilize.

Other Approaches to Antithyroid Drug Therapy

You may encounter differing methods of antithyroid drug therapy:

1.   Some doctors begin treatment with large doses of antithyroid drugs—perhaps 300–400 mg of PTU or 30–40 mg of methimazole per day—to block thyroid hormone production. These doctors also maintain the large starting dose for long-term therapy. To prevent the hypothyroidism that would certainly develop if you continued to take large doses of an antithyroid drug, these physicians also prescribe a replacement dosage of thyroid hormones as soon as you become euthyroid (see chapter 13).

If you are managed by this approach for the long term, you will be taking two different medications in full dosage.

There are several disadvantages to this approach to antithyroid drug therapy. First is the practical necessity of taking two separate medications, at more cost to you, than a maintenance dosage of antithyroid drug alone. Second, large doses of antithyroid drugs may increase the probability that you will develop significant side effects from these drugs.

2. Some doctors will begin treating a patient with an appropriate dosage of methimazole or PTU, but they will discontinue the drug as soon as the patient becomes euthyroid. A few patients may enter remission during the first several months of treatment, but most will relapse. Many such patients are then referred to an endocrinologist because of "antithyroid drug failure." There is, of course, no drug failure in this situation, only failure of the doctor to prescribe the drug appropriately. Clinical experience indicates that the longer a patient takes antithyroid drugs, the more likely the possibility of remission. Most experienced clinicians will prescribe antithyroid drugs for one or two years before evaluating a patient for remission.

Complications of Antithyroid Drugs

As is true of many other drugs, use of the antithyroid drugs PTU and methimazole is associated with side effects in some patients. About 5 percent of treated patients develop an itchy red rash that may sometimes look like hives, a low-grade fever, and mild aching in the joints. Although annoying, these side effects are not serious to your health. Your doctor may prescribe mild analgesics such as aspirin or acetaminophen to relieve your fever and the aching in your joints and an antihistamine medication such as diphenhydramine (Benadryl) or chlorpheniramine (Chlorotrimeton) for relief of itching.

These complaints often disappear spontaneously with continued use of the antithyroid drug and a brief interval of treatment with the above medications. If your symptoms are not significantly improved on this regimen, your doctor may switch from one antithyroid drug to the other. For example, if you developed a rash during treatment with methimazole, your doctor can stop methimazole therapy and begin treatment with PTU. You have better than a 50 percent chance of tolerating the alternative drug without side effects. Most of the mild side effects of antithyroid drugs develop within the first several months of treatment. If you have been taking the drugs for more than three or four months, it is very unlikely that you will develop one of these complications.

Severe Reactions

A number of severe reactions may occur during treatment with antithyroid drugs, but they are fortunately quite rare, affecting about one out of every 200 to one out of every 300 treated patients. Most common of the rare complications is the sudden loss of the white blood cells that fight infection, the granulocytes. This disorder is called *agranulocytosis*. Since a major role of granulocytes is to combat infection, patients who develop agranulocytosis usually develop an infection, commonly a sore throat with fever and, occasionally, a rash. You should be sure to stop taking the antithyroid drug immediately and to call your doctor if such symptoms or signs develop.

If you develop agranulocytosis, your doctor will probably hospitalize you so that you can receive appropriate antibiotic therapy. The number of granulocytes usually begins to rise within several days after the antithyroid drug is discontinued, but their numbers may not normalize for one to two weeks. When agranulocytosis occurs, it has a sudden onset that is only rarely predicted even by weekly or semiweekly measurement of your white blood count, so routine blood counts are unnecessary. However, if your doctor does measure your granulocyte count while you are on antithyroid drug therapy, and the count is less than 1,500 cells per cubic milliliter, it should be watched closely; the therapy will be discontinued if the count decreases further.

Several other serious reactions that occur even less frequently than agranulocytosis are a form of noninfectious hepatitis, arthritis in multiple joints, and high fever. Hepatitis will begin with yellowing of your skin and eyes. You should stop taking the antithyroid drug immediately and call your doctor if this occurs.

Like the relatively minor side effects of antithyroid drug therapy, the rare serious complications of antithyroid drugs usually show up within the first several months of therapy. They become more frequent with larger doses of drugs. If antithyroid drugs are discontinued because you develop any of these side effects, hyperthyroidism will recur and should probably be treated with radioactive iodide.

Long-Term Management

Antithyroid drugs do not cure hyperthyroidism. They control the disease while the patient and physician remain hopeful of a remission of hyperthyroidism. Some patients elect to take these drugs for lifelong therapy even if their disease does not remit.

Remission may occur at any time, from several weeks to many months after treatment has started. Most endocrinologists will maintain you on antithyroid drugs for one to two years to see if remission has occurred. If hyperthyroidism recurs after drug therapy is stopped, antithyroid drugs can be prescribed for another one to two years. If you do not have a remission after two to four years of antithyroid drug treatment, it is very unlikely that your disease will ever go into remission. You may then decide to continue with the antithyroid drugs indefinitely, at a maintenance dosage, to control the hyperthyroidism and remain in the euthyroid state.

If this is the case, you should see your doctor for a brief examination and measurement of serum T_4 and TSH about every six months. Your doctor may adjust your maintenance dosage of PTU or methimazole from time to time, based on the results of these evaluations. Alternatively, if remission does not occur, you may decide to discontinue antithyroid therapy and be treated with radioactive iodide.

Remission of Hyperthyroidism

While you are under treatment, several findings can suggest that your hyperthyroidism is in remission. If your doctor finds that your thyroid gland has significantly decreased in size during your treatment, and only a small dosage of antithyroid drug is required to control your hyperthyroidism (25–50 mg of PTU or 2.5 to 5 mg of methimazole per day), then it is likely that your disease is in remission. However, these are not failsafe predictors of remission. Similarly, no single blood test result can absolutely predict a remission.

The presence of TSAb in the blood almost guarantees that your hyperthyroidism will recur after antithyroid drug therapy is stopped. However, there is a 25 to 50 percent chance of recurrent hyperthyroidism even if TSAb has disappeared from your blood. The test to determine the presence of TSAb is costly and not reliable enough to use routinely on patients with antithyroid drugs. A number of other tests are used by some physicians to predict remission, although recent studies show that none is completely reliable.

If your doctor suggests a measurement of serum thyroglobulin, a T_3 suppression test, a thyrotropin-releasing hormone (TRH) stimulation test, or a thyroidal radioactive iodide uptake test to determine whether you are in remission, you should be aware that they will be costly and not necessarily accurate in their ability to predict remission.

If your doctor thinks that you are in remission and stops treatment with antithyroid drugs, you should be alert for the development of any symptoms of hyperthyroidism. These symptoms should be familiar to you from your previous experience (see chapter 6). If any of these symptoms develop, you should be examined quickly and have measurements of serum T_4 and TSH taken. If symptoms do not develop, you should still be examined every three months for the first year. A rise in serum thyroid hormones and a decrease in serum TSH concentration will usually be present before the development of the symptoms. If symptoms and signs of hyperthyroidism do not develop, and your serum T_4 and TSH concentrations remain normal, it is likely that you are in remission.

Recurrence

After cessation of treatment with antithyroid drugs, most recurrences of hyperthyroidism will occur within the first three to six months. Although remission may be lifelong, it is more likely that you will develop hyperthyroidism again during your lifetime than someone who has never been hyperthyroid. Clinical experience suggests that more than half of patients with Graves' disease in remission will develop recurrent hyperthyroidism within five years. Since neither you nor your doctor can ever be entirely certain when a relapse may occur, you should visit your doctor for a thyroid evaluation about once a year for the rest of your life. The examination and results of measurement of serum thyroid hormones and TSH may predict a relapse before symptoms develop and you suffer any disability. Lifelong follow-up may also detect the earliest stages of hypothyroidism, which can develop many years after remission of Graves' disease (see chapters 8 and 12).

RADIOACTIVE IODIDE

Most doctors in the United States prefer radioactive iodide for the treatment of Graves' hyperthyroidism. This is an effective and safe treatment that reverses hyperthyroidism because it decreases the number of thyroid cells, along with their ability to produce and secrete excessive amounts of thyroid hormones in response to the stimulating antibody.

Radioactive iodide became available for experimental use in the early 1940s as a by-product of the nuclear fission experiments that led to development of the atomic bomb. Since it was already clear that thyroid cells take up and retain iodide from the blood, scientists soon discovered that certain doses of radioactive iodide would accumulate in the thyroid gland and destroy thyroid cells. At the same time, however, it produced few if any changes in other organs and tissues of the body.

Soon after World War II, hospitals developed laboratories for the safe use of radioactive iodide in diagnosing and treating thyroid disease. Over the last forty years, many other radioactive by-products have entered medical practice, mainly for diagnostic procedures, and now most hospitals have a department of nuclear medicine that is responsible for the medical applications of radioisotopes.

How Does Radioactive Iodide Work?

Most people have their first experience with X rays in their dentist's office. A narrow beam of X rays generated by a dental X-ray machine is directed at your teeth and produces an image on a photographic film that is placed behind the teeth. The X-radiation has the ability to pass through your body (your cheek and gums) to produce the image of your teeth on the film. Radiation can be harmful if it is used improperly or if the dosage is too large. The X-ray machine is set to deliver just the correct amount of X-radiation to expose the film. A heavy lead apron is placed over your body, including your neck, to prevent unnecessary exposure of your organs (including your thyroid) to the X ray. The dentist or hygienist also leaves the room while the X ray is taken to avoid unnecessary exposure.

Radioactive iodide emits two distinct types of radiation—*gamma rays* (similar to X rays) and *beta rays*. Gamma rays from radioactive iodide penetrate the tissues of the neck readily, making it easy to measure, with isotope-counting machines. The same radioactive iodide is used to determine thyroidal radioactive iodide uptake (see chapter 5) and to produce thyroid scans (see chapters 10 and 16). Although gamma radiation penetrates tissues readily, it produces relatively minor damage because little is absorbed by the tissues. Therefore, gamma radiation from radioactive iodide is useful for measurement and for thyroid scans but not for treatment.

The beta rays emitted by radioactive iodide are completely different from gamma radiation because they do not readily pass through tissues. Beta rays travel only several millimeters, or about one-tenth of an inch, before their energy is dissipated and absorbed by the thyroid cells, causing variable damage to DNA (genetic material in the nucleus of each cell). All cells have the ability to repair minor damage to DNA caused by radiation, but extensive damage to DNA will usually result in death of the cell. Doses of radiation that are not large enough to cause death of thyroid cells may still cause significant damage to the DNA. This in turn prevents the cell from overproducing thyroid hormone or reproducing itself.

Fifty years of experience using radioactive iodide to treat Graves' hyperthyroidism has taught physicians how to give a dosage that safely and permanently cures the hyperthyroid state. However, this can often lead to the development of an underactive thyroid—hypothyroidism—which requires treatment with thyroid hormones (see chapters 12 and 13).

How Is It Given?

The dose of radioactive iodide that will relieve your symptoms and normalize your thyroid function is not associated with deleterious effects of radiation on other organs. Many different methods of calculating the "correct" dosage have been proposed, but no one method seems superior to another. If a small dose is given, fewer patients will be cured of their hyperthyroidism and many will require a second or even a third treatment with radioactive iodide. If an excessive dose is given, almost everyone will be cured of hyperthyroidism, but most patients will also develop hypothyroidism. Therapeutic approaches vary widely and depend on your doctor's experience and philosophy of treatment.

Restoration to a Normal State

Many endocrinologists and nuclear medicine physicians will attempt to restore a normally functioning thyroid with the least risk of hypothyroidism. The dose of radioactive iodide usually depends on the estimated size of your thyroid gland and its activity, determined by measurement of the 24-hour thyroidal radioactive iodide uptake (see chapter 5). The size of your thyroid may be estimated just by physical examination or by isotopic imaging or thyroid ultrasound. A radioactive iodide uptake test will be necessary for calculating the correct dosage of iodide because there is variation among hyperthyroid patients in the ability of the thyroid to accumulate iodide. For example, consider two hyperthyroid patients with similarly enlarged thyroid glands: One has a 24-hour radioactive iodide uptake of 50 percent, and the other has a radioactive iodide uptake of 100 percent. Twice as much radioactive iodide will be required to treat the first patient in order to deliver the same dose of radioactive iodide to the thyroid gland.

Administration and Precautions

Once the dose is calculated, it is given by mouth either in liquid or capsule form. Radioactive iodide is rather tasteless and will not be irritating to your mouth, stomach, or bowels. You should not notice any immediate change in your body after swallowing the capsules. During the first day after treatment, most of the radioactive iodide accumulates in your thyroid gland, where it begins its destructive activities. The remainder is eliminated through the kidneys into your urine. It is a good idea to drink an extra two or three 8-ounce glasses of water each day for several days after taking radioactive iodide, in order to keep urine formation greater than normal. This will ensure that your bladder will empty more frequently, limiting the exposure of your bladder to the radioactive iodide. You should also be particularly careful to flush the toilet and wash your hands after you urinate. A small amount of radioactive iodide will appear in your saliva, so you should use paper plates and cups for eating and drinking and avoid intimate contact such as kissing for the first several days after treatment.

Patients are often concerned that the radioactivity they receive from treatment with radioactive iodide may affect others in their family. After the first 24 to 48 hours, almost all of the radioactive iodide remaining in your body will be in your thyroid gland, and the radioactivity will decrease by 50 percent every five to seven days. The doses used to treat hyperthyroid patients are considered safe for those who live with you. Nevertheless, it makes good sense to limit the amount of time you spend with infants, children, and pregnant women—at least for the first week after therapy. Some doctors suggest that you sleep alone for the first several days after treatment with radioactive iodide, but there is no evidence that the radiation from your thyroid is a risk for your partner.

It may be helpful to know that the intensity of radiation decreases with the square of the distance from the radiating source. If loved ones move from three feet away from you to nine feet away, their exposure to radiation from your thyroid will decrease nearly 10 times. If you wish to be very careful after receiving treatment with radioactive iodide, remain 5 to 10 feet away from family members and friends, and their radiation exposure will be minimal.

Initial Treatment

Ideally, only a single dose of radioactive iodide will be necessary to treat your hyperthyroidism. The radiation will initially produce inflammation in your thyroid gland that disrupts its structure and causes an even greater release of thyroid hormones. Although most patients notice no immediate changes, others may experience mild tenderness of the thyroid for the first several days after treatment; this is usually relieved by one or two tablets of acetaminophen. The increased release of thyroid hormones after treatment does not cause a perceptible worsening of hyperthyroidism, except in some elderly patients (see chapter 20) or in individuals with significant heart disease. If you have heart disease or other serious medical problems in addition to your hyperthyroidism, your thyroid function should probably be normalized with antithyroid drugs before the radioactive iodide is administered. This will decrease the amount of thyroid hormone stored in your thyroid and limit its release after treatment with radioactive iodide.

Gradual Improvement

The symptoms of hyperthyroidism improve slowly after treatment with radioactive iodide. You may notice some improvement after several weeks, but one to three months are usually required for normalization of your thyroid function. In fact, the effect of a single dose of radioactive iodide may not be complete for three to six months.

Since the rate of recovery from hyperthyroidism is quite variable among patients, you should be evaluated by your doctor frequently—every three to six weeks—after taking the radioactive iodide. The evaluation should consist of a history and physical examination that focus on symptoms and signs of hyperthyroidism and hypothyroidism, as well as measurements of serum T_4 and TSH. These frequent visits during the first three to six months after treatment will enable your doctor to administer a second dose of radioactive iodide at the earliest time, should you remain hyperthyroid, or to prescribe thyroid hormone medication should you become hypothyroid.

An optimal result of treatment would be the gradual improvement in your symptoms of hyperthyroidism, disappearance of the signs of the disease upon physical examination, normalization of your serum T_4 and TSH during the first one to three months after treatment, and maintenance of normal thyroid function thereafter.

As the pattern of your individual response to radioactive iodide treatment becomes evident, your doctor may decrease the number of office visits to every two or three months, then to six months, and finally, if your thyroid function remains normal, one visit per year.

Only about 15 percent of patients require a second dose of radioactive iodide to treat their persistent hyperthyroidism. A decision for a second dose should not be made until you have been observed for two or three months after the first dose. At that point, it should be clear whether or not your hyperthyroidism is improving. Less than 5 percent of patients require a third dose of radioactive iodide.

About 20 percent of patients develop hypothyroidism, requiring treatment with thyroid hormone during the first year after radioactive iodide treatment. The incidence of hypothyroidism during the first year after treatment increases if you require a second or a third dose of iodide. Even if you are one of the patients who appear normal (euthyroid) one year after their radioactive iodide treatment, and your serum T_4 and TSH concentrations are also normal, you should still be evaluated at annual intervals; you will continue to have a 2 to 3 percent chance of developing hypothyroidism every year after treatment.

Ten years after treatment with radioactive iodide, all patients should be cured of their hyperthyroidism, and at least 50 percent will likely be hypothyroid, requiring daily thyroid hormone treatment indefinitely (see chapter 13). The high incidence of hypothyroidism after radioactive iodide treatment is due to the immediate lethal effects of radiation in some thyroid cells and interference with the ability of other cells to reproduce themselves; both lead to a progressive decrease in the number of functioning thyroid cells. In some patients, hypothyroidism may have nothing to do with the radioactive iodide treatment. Rather, it may result from the development of different antibodies that are destructive to thyroid cells (see chapter 12) or other factors common to the usual course of Graves' disease.

The many variables that can influence the thyroid gland in Graves' disease make it imperative that you have periodic evaluations by your doctor for the rest of your life, albeit at infrequent intervals. By means of the doctor's examination and results of your serum T_4 and TSH measurements, a physician should detect hypothyroidism at its earliest stages even before symptoms develop. It will then be prudent to begin appropriate treatment at that time (see chapter 12).

MYTHS ABOUT RADIOACTIVE IODIDE TREATMENT

Allergy

Many patients believe that they cannot be treated with radioactive iodide because they are allergic to iodide. These people are usually allergic to shellfish and believe that it is the iodide content of shellfish that is the offending agent. Actually, true allergy to iodide is quite rare, and the shellfish allergies of most people are probably not due to its iodide content but to other constituents. Since many foods contain traces of iodide, we all routinely consume several hundred micrograms of iodide each day without allergic reactions. The amount of iodide contained in the treatment dose for Graves' disease is usually less than 1 microgram, or less than 1/100th of your usual daily intake. Allergic reactions are therefore not likely to occur, and you can safely be treated with radioactive iodide even if you are allergic to shellfish.

Hair Loss

Many patients fear that they will lose their hair if they are treated with radioactive iodide. They have heard that hair loss occurs if the head is radiated as part of the treatment of certain brain cancers, for example. The concern is heightened because when you are hyperthyroid, you have probably already lost some hair (see chapter 6). However, because most of the radioactive iodide is either rapidly concentrated by the thyroid gland or excreted into the urine, there is very little scalp exposure and hair follicles are not adversely affected. When your hyperthyroidism is successfully treated either with radioactive iodide or antithyroid drugs, your metabolic rate will decrease to normal and normal hair growth will resume. Since hair loss in hyperthyroidism is mainly due to breaking of hairs soon after they penetrate your scalp, you will have to wait several months for your hair to grow to its previous length.

Pregnancy

Because Graves' hyperthyroidism occurs frequently in women who are planning to have children, questions are almost always raised about the effects of radioactive iodide on subsequent pregnancies. The amount of radiation exposure to the ovaries or the testes is small—similar to the radiation exposure during commonly performed X-ray procedures such as the barium enema, ordered by gastroenterologists to evaluate the large colon, or the intravenous pyelogram, done to evaluate the kidneys, ureters, and bladder. There is no evidence that children of mothers who have been treated with radioactive iodide *before* pregnancy have an increased incidence of abnormalities. If you are hyperthyroid and want to bear children, you can be assured that radioactive iodide treatment is safe, both for you and your future offspring. However, radioactive iodide treatment *during* pregnancy can have serious consequences. You should wait at least three to six months after treatment with radioactive iodide before beginning your pregnancy; this will ensure that your hyperthyroidism has been effectively treated and that you will not require a second dose of radioactive iodide.

Both antithyroid drugs and radioactive iodide will cross the placenta and affect the developing fetus. Antithyroid drugs, used very carefully, usually result in a successful outcome to the pregnancy (see chapter 18), but radioactive iodide treatment can be very dangerous. In the first weeks of pregnancy, the radioactive iodide that enters the fetal blood circulation will affect the developing fetal tissues, significantly increasing the risk for developmental abnormalities. The thyroid gland is formed early in fetal development, concentrating iodide by the eighth to tenth week. Administration of radioactive iodide after the eighth to the tenth week of pregnancy will result in a high concentration of radioactive iodide in the fetal thyroid as well as in the mother's thyroid. The fetal thyroid could be destroyed by the radioactive iodide, leading to serious consequences of fetal hypothyroidism.

You and your doctor should be certain that you are not pregnant when you are treated with radioactive iodide. If there is any possibility that you could be pregnant, a pregnancy test should be done and found to be negative before you take the radioactive iodide. Some endocrinologists even prefer to administer radioactive iodide at the time of a menstrual period in women who engage in unprotected intercourse.

Radioactive Iodide and Cancer

Concern that treatment with radioactive iodide might cause cancers of the thyroid or of other organs and tissues was expressed as soon as this treatment became available. Most physicians initially restricted its use to older patients, in particular women who were beyond the childbearing years. Fortunately, increasing experience using radioactive iodide and careful long-term follow-up studies of many thousands of treated patients have shown no increase in development of thyroid cancer, leukemia, or cancers elsewhere in the body. Most physicians have now concluded that radioactive iodide is an effective and safe treatment of hyperthyroidism for adults of all ages, even women in their childbearing years. The treatment also seems safe for adolescents. However, most children with hyperthyroidism are still given antithyroid drugs, because long-term studies of children treated with radioactive iodide for Graves' disease have not been done.

OTHER DRUG TREATMENTS

Iodide Drops

Iodide solutions have been used to treat hyperthyroidism by generations of doctors, but its use today should be very limited. Iodide is necessary for formation of thyroid hormones (see chapter 1), yet paradoxically, treatment with large amounts of iodide actually decreases the secretion of thyroid hormones in Graves' hyperthyroidism. Treatment usually consists of one of two types of iodide drops: either Lugol's solution or a solution of saturated potassium iodide (SSKI). With either preparation, two to five drops several times each day will effectively decrease thyroid hormone secretion by, as yet, an unknown mechanism. Since the drops have a bitter, metallic taste, taking them with an ounce of juice will make them more palatable.

Unfortunately, iodide is not a good long-term treatment for hyperthyroidism. Although it decreases thyroid hormone secretion within the first few days of treatment, its effectiveness gradually decreases with time and it usually becomes ineffective after two to four weeks. For this reason, iodide treatment should never be used as the primary treatment of hyperthyroidism.

If iodide drops are prescribed by your doctor, they should be part of a plan of therapy that includes either radioactive iodide, antithyroid drugs, or surgery. Some doctors prescribe iodide drops for several weeks after radioactive iodide treatment, beginning two to seven days after the treatment. Although this combined treatment may lead to a somewhat more rapid resolution of your hyperthyroidism, some patients may mistakenly begin to take the iodide drops too soon, lessening the effectiveness of the radioactive iodide. If iodide drops are mistakenly taken on the same day or before the radioactive iodide, treatment will be rendered ineffective.

When iodide drops are prescribed along with antithyroid drugs, it becomes more imperative that the antithyroid drug treatment not be interrupted. If you forget to take several doses of antithyroid drugs, thyroid hormone formation will resume and the large amount of iodide in your thyroid from the iodide drops will facilitate formation of thyroid hormone. Since this combined drug treatment does not seem to restore your thyroid function to normal more rapidly than antithyroid drugs alone, combined drug therapy should probably be avoided except in certain rare, emergency situations and during the preparation of hyperthyroid patients for surgery. Several weeks of iodide treatment seems to decrease the blood flow to the thyroid gland, resulting in less blood loss during thyroid surgery.

Beta-Blockers

Many of the clinical symptoms and signs of hyperthyroidism are similar to those produced by the administration of excessive amounts of adrenaline, or epinephrine (see chapter 6). Although the concentration of adrenaline is not raised when you are hyperthyroid, many of your symptoms related to hyperthyroidism will be relieved by decreasing any activity that stimulates the adrenalinelike effects. Adrenaline is a hormone that affects the tissues of the body by first interacting with a receptor protein on the surfaces of cells. Beta-blockers, also called *β-adrenergic antagonists,* bind to these receptors and thereby block the activity of adrenaline. Commonly used beta-blockers such as *propranolol* and *atenolol* are used for treatment of patients with heart disease and hypertension, but they are also useful for hyperthyroidism.

Treatment with propranolol (*Inderal*; 20 mg three or four times per day) or atenolol (25 or 50 mg once or twice per day) will frequently relieve your palpitations, tremors, and agitation within hours. The degree of relief for hyperthyroid symptoms that is provided by these drugs varies among patients, but almost everyone is improved. Since the beta-blockers do not remedy the actual thyroid disorder, the amount of TSAb in your blood, or the overproduction of thyroid hormones, they should not be used as primary therapy. However, they are excellent adjuncts to treatment with radioactive iodide or antithyroid drugs because your symptoms will be relieved to some extent during the one-to-two-month interval between administration of radioactive iodide or antithyroid drugs and the normalization of your thyroid hormone blood levels.

Whether you have decided to take radioactive iodide or antithyroid drugs for treatment of your hyperthyroidism, your doctor can begin treatment with beta-blockers at once, even before the other treatments are started. Propranolol or atenolol treatment can be maintained as long as your serum thyroid hormone concentrations remain elevated. The dose can be gradually decreased, and finally discontinued, when your serum T_4 is normal. Since beta-blockers may worsen bronchial asthma and certain forms of heart disease, those drugs should be used cautiously (or not at all) in people with these disorders. Make sure your physician is knowledgeable about your medical history.

SURGERY

Surgical removal of thyroid tissue was the only effective treatment of hyperthyroidism before introduction of radioactive iodide and antithyroid drugs in the 1940s. Surgeons would carry out a subtotal thyroidectomy, a procedure requiring general anesthesia that removes about 90 percent of the thyroid tissue. In the first half of the twentieth century, subtotal thyroidectomy was a risky procedure because of relatively primitive surgical and anesthetic techniques, postoperative care, and the fact that surgery was done when patients were still hyperthyroid. Today, surgery is quite safe because patients are made euthyroid with antithyroid drugs before the operation is performed and because of significant improvements in surgical and postsurgical care. Surgery is also effective and safe when hyperthyroid patients are treated with large doses of beta-blockers for several days before and after the operation.

Complications

The risks of subtotal thyroidectomy include extremely rare anesthetic and surgical accidents and a 1 or 2 percent chance of injury to the parathyroid glands and the recurrent laryngeal nerve. Because of surgical injury to the parathyroid glands, an inadequate supply of parathyroid hormone will lead to low serum calcium concentration. Unless the blood calcium level is raised to normal concentrations, patients may experience numbness and tingling sensations around the lips, mouth, hands, and feet. They may also feel a twitching of the muscles as well as muscle cramps, irritability, and even seizures.

The recurrent laryngeal nerve, located just behind the thyroid gland, is subject to occasional injury during subtotal thyroidectomy. This nerve is important for the normal function of the muscles of the larynx, or voice box, which move the vocal cords. If your recurrent laryngeal nerve is injured during thyroidectomy, you may suffer permanent hoarseness.

Subtotal thyroidectomy, however, has been largely replaced by antithyroid drugs and radioactive iodide as the primary treatment of hyperthyroidism. Injuries to your laryngeal nerve or parathyroid glands cannot occur when your hyperthyroidism is treated with antithyroid drugs or with radioactive iodide, and neither of these medical treatments requires hospitalization or general anesthesia. Thyroidectomy will also leave a permanent neck scar. Finally, the results of surgical therapy are no better than those of radioactive iodide.

Today, the few patients with hyperthyroidism due to Graves' disease who are referred for subtotal thyroidectomy fall into three general categories: (1) children or adolescents who are allergic to antithyroid drugs, or who cannot take them reliably; (2) adults who are allergic to antithyroid drugs and who are afraid to take radioactive iodide; and (3) pregnant women who must not take radioactive iodide and who are either allergic to antithyroid drugs or require a dose large enough to adversely affect the developing baby.

If you are in one of these categories and are referred to a surgeon for subtotal thyroidectomy, you should ask the surgeon about his experience and his results with the operation. Because so few people are referred for subtotal thyroidectomy today, many general surgeons have relatively little experience with this procedure. Nevertheless, many hospitals have surgeons on staff who specialize in head and neck surgical procedures; ear, nose, and throat surgeons are also sometimes experienced in subtotal thyroidectomy.

If possible, you should be treated with antithyroid drugs for a sufficient period of time to relieve the hyperthyroidism before surgery is carried out. Most surgeons usually request that iodide drops also be administered for about 7 to 14 days before surgery. If antithyroid drugs cannot be used to normalize thyroid function before surgery (because of drug allergies or time constraints during pregnancy), surgery can be safely performed after a few days of intensive treatment with beta-blockers. Beta-blockers should be administered in the hospital, under careful observation for side effects and to ensure readiness for surgery.

If you are pregnant, surgery is most safely carried out between the fourth through sixth month of pregnancy. You should expect to be in the hospital for three to seven days after the operation, and you will be out of work for two to four weeks after the procedure. Postoperatively you should be followed by your internist or endocrinologist, who will monitor both your thyroid function and your serum calcium. Thyroid hormones can be administered whenever you develop hypothyroidism (see chapter 12), and vitamin D preparations and calcium can be prescribed to raise the serum calcium to normal in the one or two percent of patients who emerge from surgery with damaged parathyroid glands (see chapter 17).

9

TREATMENT OF GRAVES' ORBITOPATHY

An ideal cure for orbitopathy has not yet been discovered. However, treatments are available to conserve or restore your vision, relieve your symptoms, improve the function of your eye muscles, and enhance your overall appearance. The available treatments include medications that can produce serious side effects, radiation therapy, and surgery. Since all have significant risks, each must be selected carefully and individualized. Close collaboration between your endocrinologist and your ophthalmologist will usually produce the best results and the least number of complications.

BEHAVIOR OF ORBITOPATHY

If you have Graves' orbitopathy—whether or not you actually have hyperthyroid symptoms—you might be worried about losing your vision and concerned about the appearance of your eyes. You will also want relief from the aching pressurelike eye pain and irritation in your eyes. Orbitopathy often becomes progressively worse for several months, stabilizes, and then improves—usually over an interval of 6 to 12 months. Since there is no way to predict whether your eyes will improve (or how much they will improve) after your orbitopathy stabilizes, initial treatment should be designed both to protect your corneas from drying and to relieve your discomfort. You should be seen by your doctor frequently and at intervals determined by the severity of the orbitopathy and by the rate of its progression. Your doctor will check both your general and color vision, determine if you have double vision, and examine your corneas.

MILD ORBITOPATHY

Most of the 50 percent of patients with Graves' disease who also have orbitopathy have a relatively mild disorder. It generally does not cause damage to the corneas, double vision, or a decrease in the sharpness of their vision.

Prevention of Dryness

Treatment should be designed to relieve your discomfort and prevent visual loss, and you should be observed to determine whether your eye disease is progressive. An important goal of therapy is to prevent drying of your corneas, a condition that can lead to irritation, ulceration, and visual loss. If your eyelids do not cover the cornea when you are sleeping, they can be taped closed with Scotch tape or adhesive tape. An eye patch can be used at night. These simple treatments will not only protect your eyes when you are asleep but will also lessen the irritated feeling in your eyes when you are awake. Artificial tears, which can be purchased over the counter in your drugstore, can be dropped into your eyes several times a day for added lubrication.

If the tissues around your eyes are especially swollen and red in the morning, you may find that sleeping with your head elevated on two or three pillows can be helpful. A diuretic (medication that facilitates fluid loss by increasing the urine volume) may be prescribed by your doctor to lessen the swelling around your eyes.

Even with mild orbitopathy, you may be very uncomfortable in rooms with bright lights or in direct sunlight. Your eyes may be highly sensitive to the wind—even the gentle breeze you create when walking. Wearing tinted glasses often helps both problems, decreasing the intensity of light and blocking the wind. Glasses fitted with side panels of cloth material or thin leather to cover the area between the frames of your glasses and your cheekbones (similar to the sunglasses worn by mountaineers) may be helpful if you have severe sensitivity to the wind.

Cosmetic Correction

If you have mild orbitopathy and you are displeased because you have a prominent stare and some swelling around the eyes, your ophthalmologist can do one of several available surgical procedures. The surgery is designed to remove the swollen, baggy tissue and decrease the opening of your eyes so that they appear closer to normal. It should be done by an experienced ophthalmologist and only at a time when your orbitopathy has definitely stabilized. A procedure done too early in the course of orbitopathy might have to be repeated if the disease continues to progress.

Ask your ophthalmologist how many similar operations

he or she has performed and what the results have been. This is a specialized area, and some ophthalmologists have little experience with this type of corrective eyelid surgery. The extent of your doctor's training and experience will often be reflected in the final result.

SEVERE ORBITOPATHY

Fortunately, severe orbitopathy is uncommon, affecting less than 5 percent of patients with Graves' disease. Several different treatments are available to help this small group of individuals, but each treatment has potentially serious complications.

Drugs

Since Graves' orbitopathy is probably an autoimmune disorder, as is the case with Graves' hyperthyroidism, it is not surprising that several drugs widely used to suppress the autoimmune response have been tried. Cyclosporine A and azathioprine, which prevent the autoimmune rejection of kidney and heart transplants, were initially reported to improve orbitopathy in small groups of patients. However, recent results suggest that the modest improvement in orbitopathy produced by these drugs is offset by serious side effects, particularly damage to the kidneys by cyclosporine A. They are not recommended for management of orbitopathy.

Glucocorticoids such as prednisone, methylprednisolone (Medrol), and dexamethasone (Decadron) are more useful than cyclosporine A or azathioprine, particularly for short-term treatment. These drugs are derivatives of cortisol, an essential hormone secreted by the adrenal gland. In high doses, they will rapidly relieve your symptoms of eye pain, swelling, redness, and tearing. If your visual acuity is impaired, treatment with high doses of glucocorticoids may lead to an improvement. Resolution of double vision is less certain with these drugs, and their effect on bulging of the eyes is often only minimal.

Side effects.   Although glucocorticoids can offer you significant relief, particularly if your symptoms are related to inflammation (redness, swelling, tearing, and eye pain), they should not be used for long-term treatment. The dosage of glucocorticoids necessary for meaningful improvement in your orbitopathy is quite large—for example, 60 milligrams or more of prednisone per day—which can produce serious side effects. If you are treated with large doses of glucocorticoids for more than a few weeks, you will gain weight and notice extra fat deposits in your cheeks, above your collar bones, and over the base of the back of your neck. You may also notice that your muscle strength is decreasing, particularly in your thighs, so that you will find it more difficult to climb stairs or rise from a squatting position. During the first months of treatment, there will be no warning signs to indicate that your bones are losing considerable amounts of calcium and phosphate, which ultimately leads to osteoporosis. However, after long-term treatment you will be much more susceptible to fractures than people who are not treated with these drugs.

Lastly, if you have mild diabetes mellitus, even a condition not requiring insulin, glucocorticoid treatment will make it much more difficult to control your blood sugar. If you are taking insulin, the dosage will likely have to be substantially raised.

You and your physician should consider these serious side effects of glucocorticoids before you embark on therapy. If you have a marked improvement in your eye symptoms after taking high doses of glucocorticoids for several days, your doctor will recommend a progressive decrease in dosage over an interval of days to weeks. This ensures that you will be treated with the lowest dose of glucocorticoid necessary to maintain improvement in your orbitopathy.

Since smaller doses of glucocorticoids are associated with fewer side effects, your doctor may be able to treat you for several months with a smaller dosage that is still sufficient to improve your orbitopathy symptoms. However, when your doctor decreases the dosage, your orbitopathy may worsen, quickly returning to its previous state.

Radiation Therapy

If your orbitopathy is severe, and low doses of glucocorticoids are inadequate to safeguard your vision, your doctor will consider two other kinds of treatment: *radiation therapy* and *orbital decompression surgery*. The first, radiation therapy, probably interferes with the autoimmune reaction behind the eyes as well as in the eye muscles, thereby leading to improvement in your symptoms of inflammation; it also will improve your vision if it has been impaired. However, there will be little improvement in the degree of protrusion of your eyes or in double vision caused by dysfunction of your eye muscles.

For successful treatment, you must find an experienced ophthalmologist and radiotherapist who uses modern equipment. Use of a machine called the linear accelerator seems to be associated with fewer complications than the older cobalt radiotherapy machines. The radiotherapist will direct the appropriate dosage of radiation to your eyes and the orbital contents but will avoid radiating the lens of your eye or your retina, the area of your eye containing the nerve cells that receive visual images. Cataracts and inflammation of the retina can occur if your lens and retina have been irradiated excessively. Radiation therapy, which will resolve the inflammation of your Graves' orbitopathy and restore your vision (previously compromised by increased pressure on the optic nerve), is delivered in multiple small doses over several weeks, often in conjunction with low doses of glucocorticoids.

After your orbitopathy has remained stable for six to 12 months, after radiation therapy and the preservation of your vision is assured, you and your doctor can consider the various surgical procedures that will improve your appearance, relieve the protrusion of your eyes, and correct your double vision. If protrusion of your eyes is not severe and you do not have double vision, you may decide to live with the changes in your eyes without further treatment or surgery. However, if your stare is prominent and your eyes are still irritated and light-sensitive, you should consider eyelid surgery to improve your appearance and relieve your discomfort. Eyelid surgery should not be expected to diminish the excessive bulging of your eyes.

Orbital Decompression Surgery

Severe bulging of your eyes can be improved only by surgically enlarging the bony orbit, giving your eyes and eye muscles more space in that part of the skull. The surgical procedures that are used are called orbital decompressions; they are actually orbital removals, since one or more of the bony walls of the orbit are surgically removed. Orbital decompression operations should be used as a last resort for severe orbitopathy, only after glucocorticoids or radiation therapy fail to relieve serious complaints or prevent visual loss. This is because the operative procedures that are used are associated with significant complications. After orbital decompression surgery, your eyes may not appear symmetrically placed, your double vision may worsen, and you may have numbness over portions of your face because of nerve damage. However, when the surgery is carefully performed, you should have significant improvement in your vision and the bulging of your eyes should certainly decrease. Ask your ophthalmologist about how experienced he or she is in doing orbital decompressions. Since your problem is not common and your own knowledge about orbital decompression surgery will be limited, you may first want to speak with several patients who have had the procedure.

EYE MUSCLE SURGERY

Double vision is an aggravating complication of Graves' orbitopathy, and it significantly compromises most activities of day-to-day life. Normal binocular vision is usually present during the early stages of orbitopathy, but double vision may develop and worsen as your orbitopathy worsens. Therefore, even if double vision is making your life difficult and is not corrected with special glasses containing prisms, you and your doctor should wait until your orbitopathy has stabilized for at least three to six months before considering corrective eye surgery. One or more operations may be required for a good result. Successful surgery should completely eliminate double vision when you are reading or when you look straight ahead, but some patients with severe orbitopathy may still have double vision when they look to the side, up, or down.

10

HYPERTHYROIDISM DUE TO NODULES

When your hyperthyroidism is due to single or multiple lumps or nodules in your thyroid, the condition is known as *toxic nodular goiter*. "Nodular goiter" refers to the fact that your thyroid is not only enlarged but that nodules, or lumps, are present. "Toxic" is medical terminology indicating an overactive thyroid or hyperthyroidism.

DIFFERENCES BETWEEN TOXIC NODULAR GOITER AND GRAVES' DISEASE

Several important features distinguish toxic nodular goiter from Graves' disease, the most common cause of hyperthyroidism. In Graves' disease, the thyroid cells are normal and are appropriately overproducing thyroid hormones in response to the abnormal stimulator, TSAb (see chapter 7). After disappearance of TSAb, the function of your thyroid gland will return to normal, as is the case when you are in remission. TSAb is not found in patients with toxic nodular goiter, nor are other substances that stimulate thyroid cells to overproduce thyroid hormones. Exophthalmos, which commonly occurs in Graves' disease (see chapter 7), is also not found in toxic nodular goiter.

In toxic nodular goiter, the abnormality is confined to the groups of abnormal thyroid cells that overproduce thyroid hormones, resulting in increased levels of thyroid hormones in the blood. The patient will also show signs and symptoms of hyperthyroidism. Because serum TSH from the pituitary is decreased by the overproduction of thyroid hormones, the normal thyroid cells suffer from lack of stimulation and stop producing thyroid hormones. Since the abnormal thyroid cells that overproduce thyroid hormones do it "on their own" and are not dependent on TSH, their function is *autonomous*.

On examination, your doctor may feel these groups of abnormal, autonomously functioning cells as either one lump in your thyroid (a *single* or *solitary* nodule) or as multiple lumps *(multinodular goiter)*. These findings are very different from the uniform thyroid enlargement that occurs in Graves' disease (see chapter 7).

How It's Discovered

Because the autonomously functioning thyroid tissue grows very slowly, you may never develop symptoms or signs of an overactive thyroid. You may feel or see an unusual protrusion in the lower portion of the front of your neck, a friend may point it out to you, or your doctor may discover it during a routine physical examination.

Physical Examination

Any abnormality you discover in your neck area should be brought to the attention of your doctor. After taking a complete history and examining you for signs of thyroid malfunction, your physician will have blood drawn for measurement of your thyroid hormones and TSH levels. If you have nodules in your thyroid and signs of hyperthyroidism are found on examination, and if concentrations of serum thyroid hormones are increased and serum TSH decreased to less than 0.1 μU/ml, you have hyperthyroidism that is almost certainly due to overproduction of thyroid hormones by thyroid nodule(s).

If, however, there are no symptoms of hyperthyroidism, and laboratory results are within normal ranges at the time your nodule(s) are discovered, your doctor will then order a radioactive iodide scan to determine the function of your thyroid nodules. The function of your nodule(s) is an important determination because nodules that accumulate radioactive iodide poorly, compared to normal thyroid tissue, are associated with a significant risk for thyroid cancer (see chapter 17). On the other hand, nodules that accumulate radioactive iodide better than normal thyroid tissue almost never contain thyroid cancer.

Thyroid Scan

The thyroid radioactive iodide scan is an extension of the radioactive iodide uptake test (see chapter 5). After the radioactive iodide uptake is measured, a picture using a camera with film sensitive to gamma rays is developed showing how the radioactive iodide is distributed within the thyroid gland. If your thyroid gland is normal, the scan will show uniform distribution of the radioactive iodide throughout your thyroid (Figure 10.1). If you have Graves' disease (see chapter 7), the

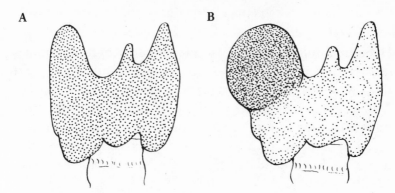

Figure 10.1. Thyroid iodide scan

A. *Normal:* Radioactive iodide, illustrated by the dots, is distributed uniformly and symmetrically throughout both lobes of the thyroid gland.
B. *Functioning thyroid nodule:* Radioactive iodide is concentrated in a nodule located in the right lobe of the thyroid gland, which corresponds to a lump felt by the doctor. Normal thyroid tissue contains little radioactive iodide, indicated by fewer dots.

scan will usually show an enlarged thyroid gland with an increased but uniform distribution of the radioactive iodide. However, if you have autonomously functioning thyroid nodules, the scan will show an increase in the radioactivity over each of the nodules, more or less proportional to their size. The nodules will then be described as "functioning," or "warm." The radioactive iodide uptake by the normal thyroid tissue may be less than normal or even absent, depending on how completely TSH production has been suppressed by the overfunctioning nodule(s).

Thyroid nodules determined to be functioning or warm should *not* be biopsied (see chapter 16) because the possibility that they contain thyroid cancer is very low. The designation of a warm, or functioning, nodule is also important because it alerts you to the possibility that you may eventually develop hyperthyroidism as the nodule enlarges.

Timing of Treatment

Hyperthyroidism caused by functioning thyroid nodules usually develops in middle-aged or older individuals, but the thyroid enlargement is often discovered years earlier. If your doctor determines that your thyroid nodules are functioning (warm) on a radioactive iodide scan, and you are not currently hyperthyroid, you should not receive any specific treatment but should arrange to see your doctor every six months to one year for reevaluation.

These follow-up visits should include an examination of your neck to determine whether the nodules have increased in size and a general examination to see if you have any signs of hyperthyroidism. Since nodules may preferentially make T_3, your doctor should order measurement of serum T_4 and T_3 as well as TSH.

Typically, your nodule(s) may gradually increase in size over a period of several years; this is associated with a gradual increase in serum T_4 and T_3 and a decrease in serum TSH. Most patients have no symptoms related to hyperthyroidism during this evolution from normal thyroid function to mild hyperthyroidism.

The optimal time for treatment is when serum TSH is just decreased to less than 0.1µU/ml, because when TSH decreases, the activity of the normal thyroid tissue that surrounds the nodule or is between nodules will also be decreased. If a dose of radioactive iodide is administered at this point, the radioactivity will then be concentrated in the functioning nodule and not affect the normal thyroid tissue.

If you are one of the minority of patients to have symptoms of hyperthyroidism before your nodules are discovered (see chapter 6), your doctor can determine the condition by ascertaining that your serum thyroid hormone concentrations are raised and that your serum TSH is decreased. A thyroid radioactive iodide scan should then show that all of the radioactivity in your thyroid is localized in your nodules and that your normal, TSH-dependent thyroid tissue accumulates radioactive iodide. Since you already have symptomatic hyperthyroidism, treatment should begin at once.

Treatment Choices

Since nodular hyperthyroidism is caused by overfunctioning thyroid tissue that is independent of TSH, the only treatment that will restore your thyroid function to normal is destruction of the abnormal tissue by radioactive iodide or surgical removal of the tissue. The appropriate choice between these treatments depends on your age, the size of the thyroid nodule, and the presence of other medical conditions that may make surgery more risky for you.

Surgery

If you are a young adult or in early middle age when you develop nodular hyperthyroidism, you should consider surgery as the first choice for treatment, especially if your functioning nodule is more than 3 to 4 centimeters in diameter.

Hyperfunctioning thyroid nodules are relatively resistant to radioactive iodide, in comparison to the thyroid tissue of Graves' disease, so that a much greater dose of radioactive iodide is necessary to resolve your hyperthyroidism. An effective dose will result in greater radiation exposure to your normal but currently inactive thyroid tissue and to other organs of your body. Surgery is the safer choice for younger patients.

Preparation for surgical treatment is similar to the preparation for surgical treatment of Graves' hyperthyroidism (see chapter 8), but the outcome is different. Your hyperthyroidism will be relieved within the first one to two weeks after surgery, and the hypothyroidism that frequently follows surgical treatment of Graves' disease is unusual after surgical removal of nodules. You should anticipate remaining in the hospital for two to four days after surgery and spending another week at home for recuperation. Annual follow-up visits with your doctor are advisable to determine whether you are one of the few patients who might develop hypothyroidism.

Radioactive Iodide

Radioactive iodide is generally the treatment of choice for middle-aged or older patients, and particularly for patients with multiple hyperfunctioning nodules. Determination of the dose of radioactive iodide and the guidelines for safety of family and friends are similar to those for the radioactive iodide treatment for Graves' disease.

Many doctors will restore older patients to the euthyroid state, using antithyroid drugs, before administration of a dose of radioactive iodide (see chapter 8). The hyperfunctioning thyroid tissue accumulates most of the radioactive iodide; the normal thyroid tissue between the nodules, which has become inactive because of suppressed serum TSH, receives a much smaller radiation dose.

After radioactive iodide treatment, you should notice gradual improvement in your hyperthyroidism, and this should be associated with a decrease in the size of your thyroid nodules. Hyperthyroidism should be completely resolved between three and six months after treatment, but in many patients some nodular tissue remains and can be felt either by you or your doctor. The residual thyroid tissue does not mean you will develop hyperthyroidism again.

When the hyperfunctioning thyroid nodules have been treated with an effective dose of radioactive iodide, your inactive but normal thyroid tissue will gradually begin to function normally.

Because some patients do develop hypothyroidism after radioactive iodide treatment, you should see your doctor once a year for a brief follow-up examination and measurement of serum thyroid hormones and TSH.

11

THE UNDERACTIVE THYROID: HYPOTHYROIDISM

Ellen R., 38 years old, was referred to an endocrinologist because her family doctor suspected she might be hypothyroid. Her doctor had seen her often during the previous two years for what the physician described as "nonspecific complaints." It was only when Ellen's teenage daughter developed enlargement of the thyroid that the doctor thought an underactive thyroid might be the cause of Ellen's problems.

After a medical history was taken, it seemed likely that Ellen had had symptoms of hypothyroidism for five to ten years. By her early thirties, Ellen began to notice increasing fatigue. She required more sleep than before, changes she attributed to working full-time and raising two daughters. The fatigue and sleepiness became progressively worse, and in the last three to five years Ellen also noticed that her mind seemed to be slowing down, that she was gaining weight without overeating, and that she was always cold.

As these complaints worsened, Ellen lost her job because of poor performance and eventually restricted her activities to her home. During the previous year her teenage daughter had taken over most of her household activities. Ellen's body felt "swollen and bloated," making it impossible to wear her rings, and she became severely constipated and resorted to enemas. Because of muscle cramps, she had difficulty climbing stairs and began sleeping on the couch in the living room.

On examination, Ellen had the typical features of severe hypothyroidism. Her hair was coarse and thinning, and there was puffiness around her eyes and in her hands and feet. Her voice was hoarse. Her heart rate was slow, between 50 and 60 beats per minute, and her blood pressure was above normal. Her skin was cold, dry, and scaly, and her nails were thin and broken. Her muscles ached whenever she moved her limbs. Her reflexes, when tested with a reflex hammer, were abnormal. Her thyroid gland was enlarged and very firm.

Ellen is typical of many patients—men and women—with severe hypothyroidism. Her disorder progressed so slowly that many of her symptoms were attributed to her busy schedule at home and at work and to "just getting older." Because the various symptoms of hypothyroidism are not specific for the disease, the diagnosis often is not made until the disease has progressed. By then, patients may already have suffered years of physical and social disability.

Advances in laboratory diagnosis now make it possible to detect hypothyroidism in almost all patients even before symptoms develop, and at relatively low cost. Once a diagnosis is made, appropriate treatment (see chapter 13) can prevent development of the symptoms and disability associated with this disorder. The treatment itself is inexpensive and without complications.

SYMPTOMS

Patients with hypothyroidism experience symptoms that are related to many different organ systems of the body. Because of thyroid hormone deficiency, both the metabolic rate and heat production are thereby decreased (see chapter 3), resulting in symptoms that are generally the opposite of those experienced by hyperthyroid patients.

Cold Sensitivity

If you are hypothyroid, you will be more comfortable in hot environments and less comfortable in cold weather. Although your body temperature will feel cooler than before, your temperature measured by a thermometer will be normal. Your sensation of coldness results from a decrease in your metabolic rate and heat production, which is a result of the lower levels of thyroid hormone in your blood (see chapter 3). Since heat production is decreased, your body will conserve heat by diverting blood flow away from your skin, keeping your skin cool and lessening heat loss from your skin by radiation.

If you are hypothyroid, perspiration is markedly decreased, limiting heat loss by evaporation. If your hypothyroidism is severe, you may not perspire at all, even in a hot, humid climate. You will feel much more comfortable in summer than others, and will dislike air-conditioning. In winter months, you will overdress for warmth compared to others, use more blankets at night, and turn up the thermostat.

Skin and Nails

A pale skin with a slight yellowish cast gradually develops as hypothyroidism progresses. The paleness may result from blood being diverted away from the skin to conserve heat, and also from mild anemia. The yellowish tint is due to an accumulation in the skin and blood of the pigment carotene, a natural substance in the diet that is usually converted into vitamin A. This conversion is delayed when you are hypothyroid, causing the pale yellow skin discoloration.

In addition to being cold to the touch, your skin will become dry and rough like fine sandpaper when severe thyroid hormone deficiency occurs. When you scratch your skin or scalp with your fingernails, flaking is common and a fine powdery dust may become evident. The dryness will be most apparent on your fingers and hands, where cracking of the skin may occur, and on your elbows and knees.

Your nails will also show various abnormalities as the disease progresses. Many hypothyroid patients notice that their nails are more brittle than normal and develop unsightly lines and grooves.

Your skin may also develop a thickened feeling, and some swelling (*myxedema*) may occur—particularly noticeable around your eyes, your fingers, and your legs. The fluid that accumulates is most apparent under the skin, where it produces obvious swelling, but it also occurs in many of the internal tissues of the body. When it involves the tongue, you may notice visible enlargement; in the vocal cords, the swelling causes characteristic hoarseness of your voice.

Hair

The hair follicles in your skin are also affected by hypothyroidism. As thyroid hormone deficiency becomes progressively more severe, you will first notice a coarsening of your hair, which will then become increasingly brittle. Eventually, you will lose hair, not only from your scalp but from all over your body, including your eyebrows, your armpits, your arms and legs, and your pubic area. Because loss of body hair develops at a very slow rate, it often goes unnoticed, rarely causing patients to seek medical attention.

Gastrointestinal Problems

A decrease in the activity of your intestinal tract almost always occurs when you are hypothyroid. The muscles in the walls of the normal intestinal tract work in a wavelike manner that sweeps digested food forward for absorption and eventually excretion through the rectum and anus. When you are hypothyroid, both the intensity and the frequency of these muscular contractions diminish, leading to a general slowdown in bowel function.

You may first notice dryness or hardness of your stool, and you will experience more straining during bowel movements. Eventually, true constipation develops and may be quite severe. Contractions of the large intestine may become so weak that bowel movements are impossible without enemas. Your bowels may expand to a very large size, leading to protrusion of your abdomen.

Weight

Most people have the misconception that hypothyroidism is a common cause of obesity (see chapter 21). Although hypothyroid patients usually do gain weight, the amount of the weight gain is modest in most patients, and extreme obesity is rare. An obvious cause of some of the weight gain in hypothyroidism is the extra fluid that accumulates under the skin of the legs and hands and throughout the rest of the body. A lower metabolic rate and decreasing physical activity both lead to a decrease in daily caloric requirements. Therefore, even though you may be eating less than you usually do, you may still gain a modest amount of weight as you develop hypothyroidism.

Behavioral Changes

As you develop hypothyroidism, you may experience fatigue, drowsiness, and a decreased ability to concentrate on mental or physical tasks. You may notice a mild intellectual impairment, which you may attribute to stress or fatigue. Reading and calculating will gradually become more difficult, eventually requiring a concentrated effort even for relatively simple tasks. Slowing of your mental functions, combined with a decrease in your attention span, may result in deterioration in your performance at work and in carrying out your usual daily activities.

A lack of interest in personal relationships, drowsiness, an increase in duration of sleep, slowing of speech, and generalized apathy may lead to further disability and even consideration of clinical depression as the cause of the changes.

Some psychiatrists believe that subtle forms of hypothyroidism are at the root of depression in many patients despite normal thyroid tests, and that the addition of thyroid hormones to the drug therapy of depression may facilitate recovery. Most endocrinologists, however, agree that patients who have clinical depression do not usually have hypothyroidism.

Progression of these mental and emotional changes is quite variable as the severity of hypothyroidism increases. Patients are often not aware of their impairment until after they have been appropriately treated and restored to normal thyroid function. In its most advanced form (which is rare), the impairment may be so severe that family or friends will bring the patient to the hospital because they find it increasingly difficult to arouse him or her from a stuporous condition.

Neurological Disorders

Impairment of nerves occurs in many patients with hypothyroidism, particularly in those with moderately severe thyroid hormone deficiency. Abnormal and annoying sensations, including the feeling of pins and needles, often occur in the hands and feet. A common disorder called *carpal tunnel syndrome* results in pins and needles as well as occasional cramping pain in your hands and all of your fingers except the pinkie. The symptoms are caused by excessive pressure on the median nerve, which passes from your forearm into your hand through the carpal tunnel, a small, narrow space in the front of your wrist.

When you have a carpal tunnel syndrome due to hypothyroidism or other causes, the feeling of pins and needles in your hands will often worsen at night and will be exaggerated when your doctor taps you over your inner wrist. It will feel like a mild electric shock shooting down your hands into your fingers. Since hypothyroidism is a common finding in patients with carpal tunnel syndrome, you should be evaluated for hypothyroidism if you have this condition. The syndrome will diminish and eventually disappear as your thyroid function is restored to normal by thyroid hormone treatment (see chapter 13).

You may also find that your body movements are not as fluid and coordinated as before and that you seem to be more clumsy. Your body movements may become slow and deliberate, requiring concentrated effort to accomplish relatively simple tasks such as rising from a chair or merely walking. Such changes probably reflect deficiency of thyroid hormones in the cerebellum, an area of the brain that is responsible for balance and coordination of muscle function.

Muscular Difficulties

Difficulty in carrying out simple movements may occur even when nerve function is normal because of pain in the muscles. You may feel only a vague aching discomfort in your muscles and joints, or you may have cramping pain during the night that interferes with your sleep and limits your physical activity during the day. Occasionally, patients may go to their doctors initially because they believe they have arthritis or a muscle disorder. Treatment with thyroid hormone will relieve these complaints and result in normal muscle function.

Cardiovascular Disorders

In contrast to the sudden onset of rapid heartbeat that accompanies hyperthyroidism, the heart problems common in hypothyroidism produce no alarming symptoms. A gradual slowing of your heart rate and a decrease in the amount of blood pumped during each heart contraction occurs, and this leads to an overall decrease in the amount of blood pumped out of the heart to the different organs of the body. But since decreased blood flow parallels a decrease in metabolic rate, no specific symptoms develop until hypothyroid patients begin to exert themselves.

Unlike individuals with normal thyroid function, hypothyroid patients are unable to increase the amount of blood pumped by their heart during physical exertions. Therefore, if you are hypothyroid and exert yourself physically, you will likely experience some shortness of breath and become fatigued easily, making it difficult to complete your tasks. Such symptoms will usually disappear during periods of rest.

Menstruation

When a woman is hypothyroid, her menstrual flow will not only be greater than usual and extend for a longer period of time but also may reappear between the usual menstrual periods. Underlying these changes is a failure to produce eggs on the usual monthly cycle, which results in persistent stimulation of the lining of the uterus by female sex hormones (estrogens).

Failure to produce eggs, called *anovulation*, is a common feature of hypothyroidism, and results in infertility. Women with hypothyroidism do occasionally conceive, but their pregnancies are associated with a high rate of miscarriage, stillbirth, and premature delivery.

Irregular menstrual cycles are common occurrences in women with normal thyroid function. Unfortunately, some physicians still prescribe thyroid hormone medications for the purpose of normalizing menstrual cycles. Such antiquated treatment is inappropriate unless hypothyroidism is the cause of the irregular menstrual cycles.

12

CAUSES OF HYPOTHYROIDISM

HASHIMOTO'S THYROIDITIS

Hashimoto's thyroiditis is the most common cause of hypo-thyroidism in patients who have not previously been treated for an overactive thyroid. This condition is named after the Japanese physician who first described the inflammation of the thyroid that he saw through a microscope in 1912.

If you have Hashimoto's thyroiditis, your thyroid will become infiltrated with white blood cells called lymphocytes, the cells that are responsible for immune reactions. Lymphocytes will gradually replace normal thyroid tissue, causing enlargement of your thyroid and the slow development of the symptoms and signs of hypothyroidism (see chapter 11). Scar tissue will replace the lymphocytes over the course of time, eventually leading to a small thyroid gland that may be almost unrecognizable.

What Causes It

Like Graves' disease (see chapter 7), Hashimoto's thyroiditis is an autoimmune disorder. Antibodies in your blood appear in conjunction with the thyroid inflammation. These antibodies are made in response to two thyroid antigens, or proteins, thyroglobulin and thyroid peroxidase (TPO), both critically important for normal thyroid function. Thyroglobulin is the protein within which the thyroid hormones are made, and TPO is the protein enzyme that activates iodide and inserts it into thyroglobulin (see chapter 1). Medical scientists still do not know what initially triggers the production of antibodies to these two proteins in affected patients.

If you have Hashimoto's thyroiditis, you will have an 80 percent chance of having antithyroglobulin and antithyroid microsomal (TPO) antibodies detectable in a blood test. Tests for the presence of these antibodies are straightforward and inexpensive, and they are the basis for making the diagnosis. Most laboratories will provide measurements of both antibodies when the test is requested by your physician. However, it is sufficient and less costly to measure antithyroid microsomal antibodies alone, since the presence of these antibodies occurs more frequently than antithyroglobulin antibodies in patients with Hashimoto's thyroiditis.

Relationship of Hashimoto's Thyroiditis and Graves' Disease

Although these disorders have opposite effects, with Hashimoto's causing hypothyroidism and Graves' resulting in hyperthyroidism, they seem closely related because they are both autoimmune thyroid disorders. Not only are antibodies present in both of them, but both may occur in the same family. It is not uncommon to find that a mother and one daughter have Hashimoto's thyroiditis and that two other daughters have Graves' disease, or that one identical twin has Hashimoto's thyroiditis while the other has Graves' disease.

Moreover, if you have Hashimoto's thyroiditis, you may develop hyperthyroidism due to Graves' disease. If you have untreated Graves' disease, you may eventually develop Hashimoto's thyroiditis and hypothyroidism.

Symptoms

When you have Hashimoto's thyroiditis, you will probably experience progressive worsening of the various symptoms of hypothyroidism (see chapter 11). Your doctor will find that you have cool, dry skin; that your pulse rate is slow, often less than 60 beats per minute; that you have swelling around your eyes; that your voice is hoarse and your reflexes slow. In addition, your thyroid gland may be enlarged, firm, and rubbery.

Some patients go to their doctors because of symptoms related to an enlarged thyroid—for example, a vague feeling of pressure around their throats when they wear a tight collar or when they swallow—or simply because they or others have noticed the enlargement.

Based on your medical history, your doctor will determine whether or not you have symptoms of hypothyroidism. On examination, your enlarged thyroid gland may be the only finding.

Finally, Hashimoto's thyroiditis may be discovered not because of symptoms of hypothyroidism or because you have discovered an enlarged thyroid gland but because a blood test has revealed an increase in serum TSH or the presence of antithyroglobulin or antithyroid microsomal antibodies. Depending on the stage of your disease, your doctor may or may not find that your thyroid is enlarged or that you have signs of hypothyroidism.

Diagnosis

If you have the symptoms and physical signs of hypothyroidism and an enlarged thyroid gland, it is very likely that you have Hashimoto's thyroiditis. Several simple and relatively inexpensive blood tests can confirm the diagnosis. Your doctor should order measurement of your serum T_4 and TSH. If your serum T_4 is below 5 micrograms per 100 milliliters and your serum TSH is raised above 5.0 microunits per milliliter, you clearly have thyroid glandular disease, which has caused your hypothyroidism. If your antithyroid microsomal (TPO) antibodies are present at high levels, Hashimoto's thyroiditis is the cause of your thyroid failure. This diagnostic workup should cost less than $100.

Unnecessary Tests

Unfortunately, many patients are subjected to unnecessary and expensive testing before the correct diagnosis is made. Doctors frequently order a thyroidal radioactive iodide uptake and scan, a thyroid ultrasound, and occasionally even a CT or MRI scan of the neck. These tests, which will cost over $1,000, are unnecessary and should not be done unless your doctor is concerned about the presence of thyroid cancer (see chapter 17).

If you go to your doctor because of an enlarged thyroid gland but there is no evidence of hypothyroidism either on physical examination or in laboratory measurements (normal serum T_4 and normal TSH), he or she will still suspect Hashimoto's thyroiditis on the basis of an examination of your neck.

Most patients with Hashimoto's thyroiditis have a symmetrically enlarged thyroid gland without lumps or nodules. In this instance, the thyroid will show a firm, rubbery texture, whereas most thyroid enlargements from other causes (see chapter 15) have a softer feeling on examination. Finding a significant concentration of antithyroid microsomal (TPO) antibodies in your blood serum proves that Hashimoto's thyroiditis is the cause of the thyroid enlargement and rules out the need for further testing.

Hashimoto's Disease and Thyroid Cancer

Often in the case of Hashimoto's thyroiditis, some doctors may not appreciate how firm your thyroid may feel and will be concerned that you have thyroid cancer. They will order a number of tests, including a thyroid radioactive iodide scan, ultrasound, and fine-needle aspiration biopsy of your thyroid (see chapter 17).

Although thyroid cancer may occur occasionally in patients with Hashimoto's thyroiditis, the risk of cancer is not greatly increased in this autoimmune disease. Therefore, a scan and/or biopsy should be done only if antithyroid microsomal (TPO) antibodies are not detected, if there is no apparent cause for the firm thyroid enlargement, or if there is a particularly hard area within your thyroid. Fine-needle aspiration biopsy in particular is *not* part of the routine evaluation of patients with Hashimoto's thyroiditis.

Treatment for Hashimoto's Disease

If you have the symptoms and physical signs of hypothyroidism as well as a firm thyroid enlargement, there is little question that you should be treated with thyroid hormones (see chapter 13). Hashimoto's thyroiditis with hypothyroidism disappears spontaneously, without specific treatment, in less than 10 percent of the cases.

Treatment with an appropriate dose of thyroid hormones

will restore you to normal thyroid function—the euthyroid state—relieving your symptoms and the physical signs of disease. Your enlarged thyroid gland will also decrease significantly in size, often to normal size. Occasionally, the gland may remain somewhat enlarged because of extensive scarring, but it will still be smaller than it was before treatment. With appropriate treatment, you should expect to live a normal life, free of symptoms related to thyroid disease.

There are differences in opinion about how to treat the earliest stage of Hashimoto's thyroiditis. In this stage of the disease, you will have only an enlarged thyroid gland and the presence of antithyroid microsomal (TPO) antibodies, but you still have about a 15 to 25 percent chance of developing symptoms and signs of hypothyroidism in the future. Some doctors may recommend treatment with thyroid hormone, while others prefer no specific treatment other than watchful waiting.

In most patients the disease may remain unchanged for many years. In some persons, the thyroid may decrease in size; in others, the thyroid increases in size, and hypothyroidism will eventually develop.

Treatment for Mild Hypothyroidism

If you are one of those patients whose mild hypothyroidism is diagnosed only by means of blood tests, you can be reasonably certain that your hypothyroidism will eventually become severe enough to cause symptoms and disability. It would seem prudent, therefore, for you to begin treatment with thyroid hormones now, so that you can avoid subsequent disability.

Whether or not you are treated with thyroid hormones, you should remain under medical observation, seeing your doctor at yearly intervals for the rest of your life so that any future development of thyroid dysfunction will be detected at an early stage.

THYROID SURGERY

If you have had thyroid surgery, your chances of developing an underactive thyroid will depend on the nature of the surgery and the experience of your surgeon.

Total Thyroidectomy

If your thyroid gland has been completely removed (total thyroidectomy) as a result of thyroid cancer (see chapter 17), you will require lifelong treatment with an appropriate dosage of thyroid hormone to avoid hypothyroidism.

Hemithyroidectomy

If you've had a single thyroid lobe removed (*hemithyroidectomy*) because of benign thyroid growths or in order to cure hyperthyroidism caused by hyperfunctioning nodules, you will probably not develop hypothyroidism.

The remaining thyroid lobe will generally enlarge by a process called hypertrophy, so that it can produce sufficient amounts of thyroid hormone for normal thyroid function. However, depending on the cause of the thyroid abnormality (usually a nodule) that resulted in surgery, many doctors recommend treatment with thyroid hormones to possibly prevent the formation of additional nodules in the remaining tissue (see chapter 13).

Subtotal Thyroidectomy

If you are one of the small minority of patients with Graves' disease who require surgical treatment (see chapter 8), your surgeon will usually perform a subtotal thyroidectomy, in which most of both thyroid lobes are removed. The chances of your developing hypothyroidism within the first month or two after surgery varies from 15 to 50 percent, depending on the experience of your surgeon.

Even if you have normal thyroid function after surgery, you should still see your doctor at six-month or yearly intervals. This is because a certain number of patients will develop hypothyroidism each year after subtotal thyroidectomy for Graves' disease.

Radiation Therapy

Destruction of the thyroid gland by radiation is an important cause of hypothyroidism. Radioactive iodide is used widely in the treatment of hyperthyroidism due to Graves' disease or overactive nodules. External radiation, employed in the treatment of tumors of the head and neck and in Hodgkin's disease, can also cause hypothyroidism.

If you have been treated with radioactive iodide, you have a 10 to 30 percent chance of developing permanent hypothyroidism two to six months after the treatment. If that happens, you will require lifelong treatment with thyroid hormones.

Even if your thyroid function was initially normalized by treatment with radioactive iodide, you will remain at risk for development of hypothyroidism. Two to 5 percent of patients will develop hypothyroidism each year after treatment, and after 10 years at least half of all treated patients will become hypothyroid and need to take thyroid hormone medication for the rest of their lives (see chapter 8).

Although most doctors know that hypothyroidism frequently develops after radioactive iodide treatment, many are not aware that it can develop after external radiation therapy for tumors of the head, neck, and spine. The thyroid gland is often in or at the edge of the area being radiated and may therefore receive a damaging dosage of radiation. Hypothyroidism develops in 25 to 50 percent of such patients, mostly within the first five years after treatment. If you have received radiation treatment for one of these conditions, you should be checked every six to 12 months for the development of hypothyroidism.

Iodide Deficiency

It is paradoxical that iodide, which is an essential component of thyroid hormones, can also cause the thyroid to malfunction. Your thyroid gland has evolved special biochemical processes that allow you to maintain normal thyroid function even when your diet contains either too little or too much iodide (see chapter 1). However, in those areas of the world with extreme iodide deficiency, even these adaptive mechanisms will not prevent hypothyroidism. On a worldwide basis, hypothyroidism due to extreme iodide deficiency is probably the most common thyroid disease, but in developed countries, supplementation of salt and some food products with small amounts of iodide has virtually eliminated iodide deficiency and related hypothyroidism.

Excess Iodide Intake

Living in developed countries places you at greater risk for thyroid dysfunction caused by *excessive* amounts of iodide, essentially a man-made condition. In the past, doctors prescribed iodide with various cough mixtures and expectorants, but this practice has almost disappeared as more effective drugs have been developed. Several prescription cold or sinus medications (see Table 12.1) that contain large amounts of iodide are still available, however, and should not be used if you have thyroid disease.

Currently, the most common source of excess iodide is the contrast material that is injected by radiologists during such diagnostic tests as coronary angiograms (X rays of the arteries of the heart) and intravenous pyelograms (X rays of the kidneys and bladder). Contrast material is also often injected during CT scans to provide more information about the presence of tumors or other abnormalities. The chemical compounds in contrast material contain large amounts of iodide, which is slowly released into the body for several days to several months, depending on the specific contrast agent used.

Your thyroid gland will readily adapt to the presence of large amounts of iodide, maintaining normal thyroid function so long as you do not have an underlying thyroid disease. If, however, you have Graves' disease or nodular goiter, you may develop hyperthyroidism after exposure to large amounts of

TABLE 12.1
Drugs Containing Large Amounts of Iodide

Expectorants	Iodide Products	Antiasthmatics	Cardiac Medication
Iophen	Potassium	Mudrane	Amiodarone
Organidin	iodide	tablets	
Par Glycerol	SSKI	Theophylline	
R-Gen	Pima	KI Elixir	
	Iodo-niacin	Elixophyllin-	
	Lugol's	KI Elixir	
	Solution	Iophylline	
		Elixir	
		Ornade	
		Quadrinal	
		tablets	

iodide, even if you currently have normal thyroid function (see chapter 10).

If you have previously been treated with radioactive iodide, have had thyroid surgery, or have underlying Hashimoto's thyroiditis, even with normal thyroid function, you will likely develop hypothyroidism soon after you receive a large dose of iodide.

Diagnosis and Treatment

After exposure to excessive iodide, hypothyroid symptoms such as fatigue, sleepiness, cold sensitivity, swelling in the eyes and hands, and constipation will develop rapidly over the course of several weeks.

Your doctor will find typical signs of hypothyroidism during the examination, and the diagnosis of hypothyroidism is easily confirmed by measurements of blood levels of T_4 and TSH. Once the diagnosis is made, your doctor should determine the underlying cause of your thyroid disease, if it has not previously been established.

If you have not previously been treated with radioactive iodide or have had thyroid surgery, you will likely have Hashimoto's thyroiditis, which can be easily determined by measurement of antithyroid microsomal (TPO) antibodies. Expensive diagnostic tests such as radioactive iodide uptake and scan, thyroid ultrasound, and CT or MRI scans of the neck are rarely necessary to establish the diagnosis. Treatment with thyroid hormone will then rapidly reverse your symptoms, restoring you to normal thyroid function.

Lithium

Lithium carbonate, a drug that is widely used for the treatment of psychiatric disorders, has multiple effects on thyroid hormone synthesis and secretion, resulting in thyroid enlargement in many patients, inapparent hypothyroidism in 20 to 30 percent of patients, and symptomatic hypothyroidism in 10 to 20 percent of patients who must take this drug.

The development of hypothyroidism is usually gradual, and symptoms are often overlooked both by patients and their doctors. If you know you have thyroid disease, and you must begin treatment with lithium, you should be closely observed for development of hypothyroidism. In the absence of known thyroid disease, baseline thyroid function tests should be performed and you should be monitored for thyroid dysfunction several times during the first year of lithium treatment and yearly thereafter. If hypothyroidism does develop during lithium therapy, thyroid hormone treatment should be added in order to restore you to a normal thyroid state.

Amiodarone

Amiodarone (*Cordarone*) is a lifesaving drug for some patients who have dangerous abnormal heart rhythms. The number of people who are treated with amiodarone is small, but the incidence of thyroid dysfunction in this group is high.

If you must be treated with amiodarone, your doctor will perform a careful thyroid examination and measurement of serum T_4 and TSH *before* drug treatment is started. This is necessary in order to compare your thyroid function before and during treatment with amiodarone.

If you have previously been treated with radioactive iodide, have had thyroid surgery, or have underlying Hashimoto's thyroiditis, you have a high risk for developing hypothyroidism during the first year of treatment with amiodarone. Since the function of your heart is profoundly affected by changes in your thyroid, you and your doctor should be alert for changes in thyroid function after treatment with amiodarone.

You should be examined and have measurements of serum T_4 and serum TSH after one month of treatment. If thyroid dysfunction does not develop, measurements every six months thereafter are adequate. If hypothyroidism does develop, thyroid hormones should be carefully added to your treatment to restore and maintain a normal thyroid state.

PITUITARY DISEASE

Hypothyroidism due to TSH deficiency is an uncommon cause of hypothyroidism, accounting for less than 5 percent of patients. However, it is extremely important to recognize this form of hypothyroidism because it results from disorders of the pituitary or hypothalamus that cause a decrease in TSH secretion.

These disorders frequently include tumors that destroy most of the pituitary. The hypothyroidism therefore may be associated with decreased function of other glands controlled by the hypothalamus and pituitary, in particular the ovaries or testicles and the adrenal cortex (see chapter 5). In the presence of decreased pituitary function, treatment with thyroid hormones alone to restore normal thyroid function may precipitate a dangerous condition of adrenal insufficiency.

Symptoms

If you have hypothyroidism due to TSH deficiency, you may develop the usual symptoms of hypothyroidism, but there may be associated symptoms related to decreased function of the sex glands and the adrenal glands.

In menstruating women, periods may gradually decrease in frequency and eventually stop, sexual desire may decline, and hair under the arms and in the genital area may become sparse. In men, impotence or infertility may occur.

When you have decreased function of the adrenal glands, you may experience a number of symptoms: exhaustion; light-headedness after changing to an upright position, which is due to a temporary fall in blood pressure; and feelings of hunger, anxiety, and perspiration several hours after you eat, a result of a drop in blood sugar. You may also develop symptoms such as headache and visual disturbances, which are directly related to a pituitary or hypothalamic tumor (often the cause of TSH deficiency, and resultant hypothyroidism).

Diagnosis

Your doctor will find signs of hypothyroidism on physical examination and will order determination of your serum T_4 and TSH levels. Your serum T_4 will be decreased to less than 5 μg/dl, and your serum TSH will be either undetectable or, paradoxically, within the normal range. Many doctors do not know that patients who are hypothyroid because of failure of pituitary function will often have a normal serum TSH. This is because of the presence of abnormal TSH molecules in the blood. Although these have little or no ability to stimulate the thyroid gland, they are detected in laboratory tests and reported as normal TSH.

If you have hypothyroidism confirmed by a decrease in serum T_4, and your serum TSH concentration is not increased to more than 5 μU/ml, your hypothyroidism is likely caused by a disease of your hypothalamus or anterior pituitary. Once this is recognized, your doctor will test for other glandular functions regulated by the pituitary, check gonadal and adrenal function, and carry out a CT scan or an MRI of the brain focusing on the hypothalamic and pituitary areas looking for the cause of the problem.

Treatment

Treatment of your hypothyroidism should begin only after the full extent of your glandular deficiencies is defined. If it is established that you have decreased adrenal function in addition to hypothyroidism, you should be treated with a glucocorticoid hormone, such as cortisol, together with thyroid hormones. Thyroid hormone treatment alone should be given only if it is clear from the various tests that your adrenal function is normal. Further treatment of the specific hypothalamic or pituitary disease that has caused a decrease in TSH secretion will depend on the nature of the specific illness.

13

TREATING HYPOTHYROIDISM

The specific symptoms of severe hypothyroidism were first linked to the absence of the thyroid gland about 100 years ago. Within only a few years, doctors began to treat the disease by transplanting or injecting the thyroid glands of animals (pigs or cows) directly into human patients. These initial treatments were quickly replaced by feeding animal thyroid glands to hypothyroid patients. A prescription from the early 1890s called for patients to "take half a thyroid, lightly fried and minced, to be taken with currant jelly once a week."

Tablets of dried, or desiccated, animal thyroid glands soon became available and have been used worldwide for successful treatment of hypothyroidism. Only recently have they been replaced with pure synthetic thyroid hormones.

Restoration of hypothyroid patients to a normal, or euthyroid, state by means of thyroid hormone therapy is one of the great achievements of modern medicine, and it has benefited many millions of patients.

WHICH DRUG SHOULD BE USED?

A confusing array of thyroid medications is available to treat your thyroid hormone deficiency and maintain you in a normal euthyroid state. These include dried animal thyroid glands and animal thyroid extracts, synthetic thyroxine (T_4), synthetic triiodothyronine (T_3), and tablets that contain both synthetic thyroxine (T_4) and triiodothyronine (T_3) in different ratios of one to the other.

The drug of choice, however, is synthetic L-thyroxine. About 20 years ago, researchers discovered that the normal thyroid gland secretes mainly thyroxine and that most T_3 in your body is produced in the liver by the removal of an iodide atom from T_4 (see chapter 1). Therefore, it seems only logical that the best way for your doctor to simulate normal thyroid function when you are hypothyroid is to administer synthetic L-thyroxine and allow your body to generate T_3 naturally.

If you are treated with an appropriate dosage of L-thyroxine, your serum TSH will be normalized. Your serum T_4 and T_3 concentrations will also be raised into the normal range and remain relatively constant throughout the day, similar to those with normal thyroid function. In this way, you will be restored to normal thyroid function.

All of the available thyroid hormone medications can restore normal thyroid function and normalize your serum TSH, but only L-thyroxine treatment will result in serum thyroid hormone concentrations that most nearly replicate those of normal individuals. L-thyroxine has thus become the most widely prescribed of the thyroid medications.

Brand Name versus Generic Medication

Several brand-name products and a number of generic preparations of L-thyroxine are marketed for patients with hypothyroidism. Theoretically, all preparations, whether brand or generic, should satisfy the requirements of the Food and Drug Administration (FDA) for potency, stability, and effectiveness.

Generic preparations have the advantage of being much less expensive than brand-name products because most companies that produce generic compounds invest much less money in research, development, and promotion through packaging and advertising. Because of lower costs, government agencies and medical insurance plans promote the use of generic medications, including L-thyroxine.

All of these potential advantages of generic L-thyroxine preparations are offset by one significant factor. Although recent studies indicate that most generic preparations of L-thyroxine contain the designated amount of the drug, occasional preparations contain less than the stated amount of the synthetic hormone.

Since you cannot know in advance which generic preparation you will receive from your pharmacist, and since your pharmacist cannot know which generic preparation may have a decreased content of L-thyroxine, you will always be at some small risk for development of hypothyroidism when you start a new bottle of generic L-thyroxine. It is for this reason that many physicians prescribe one of the brand-name preparations—*Synthroid, Levothroid, Levoxine,* or *Levo-T*—to be more certain that you receive a reliable preparation. But even different brands may not be interchangeable.

The cost can vary between $15 and $30 for a three-month supply.

Dosage

The dose of L-thyroxine prescribed by your doctor depends on your age, your body size, and whether or not you have other illnesses in addition to your hypothyroidism.

If you are young, have an average body size, and have no other significant illnesses, your doctor may prescribe 0.1 mg* per day of L-thyroxine, a dose that may be sufficient to restore normal thyroid function.

If you have heart disease in addition to hypothyroidism or if you are middle-aged or older (a time of life when underlying heart disease could be present), your doctor should prescribe a much lower initial dose of L-thyroxine, about 0.025 to 0.05 mg* per day.

A larger initial dose of L-thyroxine may raise your metabolic rate more quickly than your heart can respond to the increased demand for blood. Chest pain may result, because the arteries that carry blood to the heart may be narrowed by arteriosclerosis.

Raising the metabolic rate slowly, which occurs when you start taking a smaller dosage of L-thyroxine, is generally safe. Your dosage can then gradually be raised to a level that relieves your hypothyroid symptoms—over the course of several months.

Establishing a Lifelong Routine

L-thyroxine, which is made in tablet form, can be taken at any time during the day, before or after meals. Since most causes of hypothyroidism are not reversible, you will probably continue to take L-thyroxine for the rest of your life. Therefore, it is a good idea to develop the habit of taking the medication at the same time as you do some other routine

*These dosages are given as general guidelines only. Your physician will determine the precise dose for you after appropriate examination and testing.

daily activity, such as brushing your teeth or drinking your morning coffee. If you keep your medication next to your toothbrush or coffee cup, you will soon be taking your daily medication automatically, preventing missed doses.

If you realize that you have forgotten to take a dose of L-thyroxine, simply take two tablets the next day. Each L-thyroxine molecule remains in your body for many days, so you will not notice any immediate decline in your well-being because of a missed dose, and you can easily compensate for it by taking an extra tablet the next day.

If you are someone who often misses daily doses of L-thyroxine because you do not like the idea of taking medicine for the rest of your life, you should think of L-thyroxine more as a necessary supplement than a medication. Taking L-thyroxine is similar in some ways to taking vitamins: In both cases, daily ingestion supplements a deficiency.

Long-Term Treatment

The goal of treatment with thyroid hormones is to relieve your symptoms and normalize your serum T_4 and TSH.

Each dosage of L-thyroxine slowly enters all of the organs in your body and is then slowly eliminated. It usually takes three to six weeks of treatment before your daily L-thyroxine dose is completely assimilated by the organs of your body.

Improvement in your symptoms of hypothyroidism will be gradual, occurring over several weeks to several months after beginning treatment. Your doctor will not ask you to return for a follow-up visit until you have been treated with one dose of L-thyroxine for at least one month.

Dosage Adjustment

At your follow-up visit, your doctor will determine the extent of improvement in your symptoms, see whether the clinical signs of hypothyroidism have disappeared, and request measurement of your serum T_4 and TSH. If your symptoms are completely relieved and your serum T_4 and TSH concentrations have been restored to the normal range, your doctor will approve continued treatment with your current daily dose of L-thyroxine. You then will be asked to return for reevaluation in six months to one year. If your symptoms have not been completely relieved and your serum TSH remains above the normal range, your doctor will prescribe a somewhat larger dose of L-thyroxine.

In some instances, the initial dosage of L-thyroxine may not only relieve all of your symptoms of hypothyroidism but also result in a slight overdosage of hormone, reflected by a raised level of serum T_4 and decreased concentration of serum TSH. If this occurs, your doctor will prescribe a smaller dosage of L-thyroxine.

Once your doctor determines the dosage of L-thyroxine that restores you to a euthyroid condition and normalizes your serum TSH, that dosage will probably remain unchanged for many years. Since dosage of L-thyroxine does not often change significantly, it will not be necessary for you to see your doctor more than once each year for a brief clinical evaluation, measurement of your serum T_4 and TSH, and a new prescription for medication.

What You Should Expect from Treatment

Relief of your symptoms of hypothyroidism should occur gradually, over several weeks, and the degree of your improvement will usually be related to the dose of L-thyroxine. If you were treated initially with 0.1 mg per day (which turns out to be the appropriate dose to restore you to the euthyroid state), your symptoms of coldness, fatigue, constipation, and muscle cramps should gradually diminish and completely disappear in three to four weeks. You will continue to remain well thereafter as long as you take your daily tablet of L-thyroxine.

If your treatment was started with a much smaller dosage of L-thyroxine, the initial rate of improvement in your symptoms will be slower, with resolution of your illness occurring over months rather than weeks. Your symptoms can be relieved faster once your dosage of L-thyroxine is increased.

Most patients are gratified with the relief of their symptoms. Their energy increases and quality of life is greatly improved. Even if you had few complaints before treatment, you will probably notice a significant change for the better in your feeling of well-being and your ability to carry out your daily activities after L-thyroxine treatment.

Continued Lack of Energy

Despite significant improvement, some patients continue to complain of lack of energy and the inability to lose weight despite taking a dose of L-thyroxine that restores their serum T_4 and TSH to normal. They often urge their doctor to prescribe a larger dose of L-thyroxine.

Your serum TSH concentration is the most sensitive measure available of the effects of thyroid hormone in your body. So if your serum TSH has been decreased to normal values during treatment, your doctor will conclude that your current dosage of L-thyroxine is appropriate for you and that your lack of energy and inability to lose weight must be due to other factors.

Your doctor should then carry out a complete examination, with various blood tests to determine the cause of your complaints.

Effects of Underdosage

If your dose of L-thyroxine is not sufficient to restore you to normal or if you frequently forget to take your medication, you may continue to experience symptoms of hypothyroidism, such as mild fatigue, that can impair daily functioning.

Even hypothyroidism that is so mild that it does not produce noticeable symptoms may result in hypertension and an increase in serum cholesterol. Both are risk factors for development of heart disease. You can easily avoid these problems by reliably taking the proper dosage of L-thyroxine, with minimal medical follow-up and occasional measurement of serum TSH.

Effects of Overdosage

If your dosage of L-thyroxine is too high, it will result in a cure of your hypothyroidism but also in the development of hyperthyroidism, documented by decreased serum TSH. You will therefore be at increased risk for development of sudden abnormal rhythms of the heart, very rapid heartbeat, and possibly the loss of calcium from your bones.

It has been known for many years that patients with severe hyperthyroidism have a loss of calcium in their bones, and some recent reports indicate that patients taking a dosage of L-thyroxine that decreases serum TSH to below the normal range may also have decreased calcium levels. Although it is not certain that long-term treatment with an excessive dosage of L-thyroxine leads to loss of bone density (osteoporosis) and an increased risk of fractures, these potential problems can be avoided simply by taking no higher a dosage of L-thyroxine than is necessary to restore your thyroid function to a normal state.

Allergies and Side Effects

Because the L-thyroxine you take as medication is chemically identical to the L-thyroxine manufactured by your body, it does not cause allergic reactions, stomach upsets, headaches, skin rashes, or any other symptoms—so long as the prescribed dosage is sufficient to restore you to the normal (euthyroid) state.

Interactions with Other Medications

Doctors will always ask you if you are taking other medications before they prescribe L-thyroxine. Since thyroid hormones regulate the metabolism of many drugs (see chapter 3), drug metabolism will be slowed when you are hypothyroid but will return to normal during L-thyroxine treatment. Therefore, the dosage of other medications (such as anticoagulants) that were suitable when you were hypothyroid may be inadequate after you are restored to the euthyroid state. Your doctor will decide whether the dosages of your other medications will need to be adjusted once L-thyroxine treatment is started.

Some medications, particularly the drugs used to suppress seizures, phenytoin (*Dilantin*) and carbamazepine (*Tegretol*), can increase the rate at which L-thyroxine is metabolized and thereby reduce the benefit of L-thyroxine treatment. If you begin to take one of these anticonvulsant medications, your daily dosage of L-thyroxine will probably need to be increased.

A class of drugs that bind bile acids, colestipol (*Colestid*) and cholestyramine (*Questran*), is used to decrease serum cholesterol in some patients but can significantly interfere with the absorption of L-thyroxine. This problem can be simply prevented by taking the two medications at different times.

You should take your L-thyroxine tablet on arising, followed by your first dose of bile acid resin several hours later.

Several other drugs may interfere with absorption of L-thyroxine and should not be taken at the same time as thyroid medication. These include ferrous sulfate, used to treat iron deficiency anemia, aluminum hydroxide, and antacid, and sucralfate, used by patients with duodenal ulcers.

Treatment of Hypothyroidism Due to TSH Deficiency

If you are one of the few patients who have hypothyroidism due to a pituitary or hypothalamic disorder, treatment of your associated hormonal deficiencies, particularly decreased adrenal gland function, should be given together with L-thyroxine.

Treatment should relieve your symptoms, and the dosage of L-thyroxine will be based on relief of your symptoms and the rise of your serum T_4 to the midnormal or high-normal range. Since your hypothyroidism was caused by a decrease in serum TSH because of disease of the anterior pituitary or hypothalamus (see chapter 12), your serum TSH cannot be used as a guide for your hormone replacement therapy.

14

THYROIDITIS

Hyperthyroidism and hypothyroidism usually occur as distinct disorders with different causes and specific treatments. Thyroiditis (inflammation of the thyroid), however, often combines the clinical features of both conditions. (See Figure 14.1.)

Patients will first develop hyperthyroidism, then hypothyroidism, before the disease resolves itself and normal thyroid function returns. No specific treatment is available for the hyperthyroid phase; the hypothyroid stage is usually brief, requiring either no treatment or only several months of treatment with L-thyroxine.

A correct diagnosis of thyroiditis will prevent inappropriate treatments (and perhaps side effects) of the hyperthyroid phase of the illness, and could also avoid unnecessary long-term treatment of the hypothyroid phase with thyroid hormones.

SUBACUTE THYROIDITIS

What Causes It

When you have subacute thyroiditis, the inflammation of your thyroid gland is caused by a viral infection. It is likely that you either currently have a viral illness or recently have had one. Many different viruses have been implicated in subacute thyroiditis, including mumps, measles, and influenza, but the usual culprits are viral infections that produce sore throat, fever, muscle aches and pains, and weakness that persist for several days before gradually improving.

Neck Pain

The most striking feature of subacute thyroiditis is thyroid pain and tenderness, which occurs in at least 90 percent of patients. The intensity of the thyroid pain varies from mild to severe. You may experience only a vague aching in the lower portion of the front of your neck, which may worsen when you swallow or turn your head from side to side. You may discover that your thyroid is tender to the touch when you press in with your fingers over the thyroid area.

Many patients initially think that their discomfort is caused by a sore throat, but the mild pain of thyroiditis is always on the outside of the throat; it lacks the dryness and raw feeling on the inside of the throat that occurs when you have a cold.

The pain of subacute thyroiditis can be excruciating, aggravated by turning your head or swallowing. It tends to shoot up from the thyroid area along the sides of your neck to the back of your jaws and into your ears. Although the pain sometimes affects only one side of the face, it may be worse at the back of your jaw or in your ears than in the neck, making you think that you have a dental problem or an ear infection. The severe pain that occurs in some patients with subacute thyroiditis may be disabling, preventing them from working and carrying out their other daily activities.

On examination, your doctor will find that your thyroid gland is extremely tender, indicating the likely cause of your problem.

Symptoms of Hyperthyroidism

Because your thyroid gland is acutely inflamed by viral infection, thyroid hormones stored in the protein thyroglobulin (see chapter 1) leak out into the circulation, unregulated by thyroid-stimulating hormone (TSH). This leakage of thyroglobulin results in excessive thyroid hormone concentrations, which lead to the symptoms of hyperthyroidism (see chapter 6): palpitations, nervousness, excessive perspiration, and weight loss.

Diagnosis

Your doctor will suspect that you have subacute (viral) thyroiditis because of your thyroid pain and the tenderness over the front of your neck. Another indication would be signs of hyperthyroidism that, upon examination of the thyroid, are not typical of common causes such as Graves' disease and nodules.

A diagnosis of hyperthyroidism will be easily confirmed by finding an increase in concentration of your serum T_4 or free T_4 and a decrease in your serum TSH to <0.1 μU/ml (see chapter 5). Because you will not have the characteristic eye disorder of Graves' disease, your doctor will then order measurement of your thyroidal uptake of radioactive iodide to determine the cause of your hyperthyroidism.

With thyroiditis the inflamed gland is unable to concen-

Hyperthyroidism

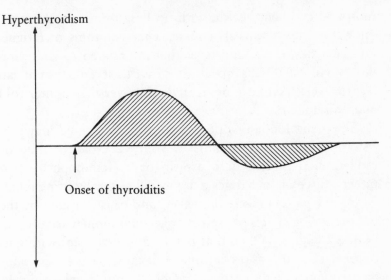

Onset of thyroiditis

Hypothyroidism

Figure 14.1. Clinical progression of thyroiditis. At the beginning of thyroiditis, patients may develop hyperthyroidism, which may persist for one to three months. This may be followed by hypothyroidism, which may also persist for one to three months before normal thyroid function is restored.

trate the radioactive iodide and the thyroid radioactive iodide uptake will be low or even zero, just the opposite of what occurs in Graves' disease or nodular hyperthyroidism. So, paradoxically, although your thyroid function is decreased, the blood tests are characteristic of hyperthyroidism. It is the unregulated release of thyroid hormones from your inflamed thyroid gland, manufactured and stored before your viral illness developed, that causes your hyperthyroidism.

Treatment

When you have thyroiditis, you can expect some disability that may persist from six to twelve months, but you will return to excellent health, with no long-term consequences, after the disease runs its course. The symptoms of fatigue, muscle aches, chills, and fever that are related to your viral illness will usually disappear after four to seven days but can last for weeks, and can be treated with over-the-counter cold and flu remedies.

The painful inflammation of your thyroid gland may persist for one to three months. If your neck pain is mild or moderate, treatment with aspirin or acetaminophen—two tablets, three or four times a day—will generally bring relief.

If your pain is severe, however, and causes disability, the pain-relieving effects of aspirin or acetaminophen usually will not be adequate. When that is the case, treatment with glucocorticoids, such as prednisone or dexamethasone (see chapter 9), will provide dramatic relief of your pain within 24 hours. The medication should be taken at the lowest dosage that relieves your pain, and continued for four to six weeks after your pain has disappeared, before it is gradually withdrawn. More than 90 percent of affected patients remain free of pain during and after this treatment.

Glucocorticoids will be prescribed as a last resort, only after treatment with aspirin or acetaminophen has failed to decrease your pain to a tolerable level. This is because the large doses of glucocorticoids that are necessary to resolve the pain of subacute thyroiditis are associated with significant side effects such as stomach ulcers and loss of bone mass (see chapter 13). A good guide for glucocorticoid therapy is to take these drugs only when necessary and to use the smallest dosage that relieves your pain for as brief a period of time as possible.

The Hyperthyroid Phase

You can expect that the hyperthyroidism that occurs because of thyroiditis will resolve spontaneously in one to three months without any specific treatment—perhaps a little sooner if you are being treated with glucocorticoids. The duration and severity of your hyperthyroid symptoms depend on the amount of thyroid hormones that was stored in your thyroid and the severity of your thyroid inflammation. (See Figure 14.1.)

If palpitations, nervousness, weight loss, and excessive perspiration cause disability, they can usually be relieved by treatment with a beta-blocker, such as propranolol (see chapter 8). As your thyroid inflammation resolves, your symptoms will gradually improve and you will return to the normal (euthyroid) state.

The Hypothyroid Phase

It is not uncommon for a hypothyroid phase to develop while your thyroid gland is healing. Although production of thyroid hormones resumes, it often does not occur at a sufficient rate to result in normal thyroid function. Therefore, mild hypothyroidism may develop, but it usually won't require specific treatment.

However, if the severity of your fatigue, muscle aches and pains, coldness, and constipation interferes with daily activities, and your hypothyroidism is confirmed by blood tests, you may be treated with small doses of L-thyroxine for several months. Withdrawal of L-thyroxine should be attempted at intervals to see if your thyroid gland has regained its capacity to manufacture and secrete sufficient thyroid hormones to maintain you in a normal (euthyroid) state without supplementation.

Without treatment, normal thyroid function is usually restored within three to six months if you have subacute thyroiditis. Since fewer than 10 percent of those affected will develop thyroid deficiency at a later time, long-term follow-up is usually unnecessary. Moreover, since your thyroid pain and the hyperthyroid and hypothyroid phases of your illness are all self-limited, the decision to treat with glucocorticoids, beta-blockers, or L-thyroxine for the different manifestations of your illness should always take into consideration the severity of your symptoms and the degree of disability. Many patients require no medication at all as the disease evolves.

SILENT THYROIDITIS (ACUTE LYMPHOCYTIC THYROIDITIS)

Self-limited hyperthyroidism followed by hypothyroidism also characterizes a disorder called *silent thyroiditis* (Figure 14.1). Although similar to subacute thyroiditis, it is not associated with pain or tenderness of the thyroid gland and clearly has a different cause.

What Causes It

Silent thyroiditis seems to be related to Hashimoto's thyroiditis (see chapter 12) because in both disorders the thyroid gland contains large numbers of immune cells, called lymphocytes. The blood also contains antibodies directed against thyroid tissue. An as yet undiscovered factor, which does not seem to be a virus, triggers a destructive process in the thyroid gland, resulting in release of excessive amounts of previously stored thyroid hormones.

Silent thyroiditis is always self-limited, with the hyperthyroid phase persisting for one to three months; the thyroid gland then evolves into a euthyroid state, with normal function, and then into a hypothyroid state, which may also persist for one to three months. Finally, normal thyroid function is restored.

Symptoms

If you have silent thyroiditis, you will first develop symptoms of mild hyperthyroidism. You may notice a rapid heartbeat, slight nervousness, a feeling of hyperactivity, some weight loss (five or ten pounds), and increased perspiration. Your doctor will find the usual signs of mild hyperthyroidism on examination (see chapter 6). In addition, your thyroid gland will be moderately enlarged and somewhat firm. Even if you do not have enlargement of your thyroid, it will feel firm, but it will not be tender.

Diagnosis

Your doctor will confirm the diagnosis of hyperthyroidism by an increase in your serum T_4 and a decrease in your serum TSH. Since orbitopathy does not occur in silent thyroiditis, the cause of your hyperthyroidism will not be apparent, so it will be necessary to measure your 24-hour thyroidal uptake of radioactive iodide.

As in subacute (viral) thyroiditis, the thyroid uptake of radioactive iodide is decreased in silent thyroiditis, indicating that your hyperthyroidism results from unregulated release of stored thyroid hormones into your bloodstream, not from overproduction and release as in Graves' disease.

Treatment

Since both the hyperthyroid and hypothyroid phases of silent thyroiditis are usually mild, your symptoms will likely be annoying but not disabling. Short-term treatment with either a beta-blocker during the hyperthyroid phase or L-thyroxine during the hypothyroid phase will depend on the degree of your discomfort.

Approximately half of patients who have silent thyroiditis will have persistent thyroid enlargement, and many eventually develop hypothyroidism. If you have had silent thyroiditis, you should see your doctor about once each year after the disorder resolves so that thyroid hormone treatment can be started for any symptoms of hypothyroidism.

15

GOITER

Goiter, one of the most common of the thyroid disorders, is simply an enlargement of the thyroid gland.

Because the thyroid is located at the front of your neck, goiters will frequently be discovered when you look into the mirror or are adjusting the collar of your shirt or blouse. You may notice that your neck size has increased because your shirts or jewelry are tight around your neck. Friends or family members may notice a swelling or an irregular appearance at the front of your neck, or your doctor may discover the goiter during a physical examination.

Goiters are not usually painful or tender to the touch, and they rarely cause difficulty in breathing or in swallowing. However, you may be aware of a feeling of fullness and a slight pressure in the front of your neck, particularly when you swallow.

DIAGNOSIS

If you discover a goiter, you should see your doctor, who will examine you to determine whether your thyroid is uniformly enlarged. This is called a *diffuse goiter*. If it contains lumps or nodules, it is known as a *nodular goiter*.

Since diffuse goiter is often the result of Graves' disease (see chapter 7) or Hashimoto's thyroiditis (see chapter 12), your doctor will ask whether you have symptoms that could be caused either by hyperthyroidism or hypothyroidism. He or she will examine you for signs of abnormal thyroid function. If you have any signs or symptoms of diffuse goiter, or if measurements of your serum T_4 and TSH show that you have either hyperthyroidism or hypothyroidism, your doctor will begin appropriate treatment.

CAUSES

Although rare in the United States and most developed nations, iodide deficiency remains the most common cause of goiter around the world, affecting many millions of people. Insufficient iodide in the diet leads to a decrease in thyroid hormone secretion, a rise in serum TSH, and subsequent thyroid enlargement.

Some goiters, particularly diffuse goiters, seem to be directly caused by increased TSH, because the thyroid will return to normal size when TSH secretion is decreased by thyroid hormone treatment (see following).

Most goiters, especially nodular goiters, probably develop because some thyroid cells divide at a more rapid rate than others. These cells may also have enhanced ability to trap iodide and make thyroid hormones. Over many years, a slightly greater rate of cell division will result in a large group of cells in one area of the thyroid that may appear as a nodule. When this process occurs in many areas of your thyroid simultaneously, the gland will gradually develop multiple nodules of varying size and function and appear as a multinodular goiter.

DIAGNOSTIC TESTS

Radioactive Iodide Scan

The 24-hour uptake of radioactive iodide (see chapter 5) is usually normal in patients with nodular goiter, but the scan will usually show that the radioactive iodide in your thyroid gland is distributed unevenly because the various nodules are functioning differently.

The thyroid radioactive iodide scan can be useful in nodular goiter to detect an area or areas of your thyroid that concentrate more of the radioactive iodide than the rest of the gland. Those iodide-concentrating areas raise the possibility that they are autonomous and may eventually cause hyperthyroidism (see chapter 10).

Conversely, the thyroid scan may show an area that concentrated very little radioactive iodide. These are called "cold" areas on the thyroid scan, and they often can be correlated with a palpable nodule, the so-called "cold nodule" (see chapter 10).

Since thyroid cancers concentrate iodide poorly or not at all, cold nodules have an increased risk (about 5 to 15 percent) of containing thyroid cancer. Therefore, if you have a nodular goiter and your thyroid scan shows a large cold area that corresponds to a large nodule, your doctor will be suspicious. You should also be examined by an endocrinologist and possibly have a thyroid aspiration biopsy (see chapter 16) to determine the nature of the tissue within the "cold area."

Thyroid Ultrasound

The thyroid ultrasound is the most sensitive and least expensive test to outline the structure and size of the thyroid gland. A hand-held device is placed on your skin and moved around over the area of your thyroid gland. Ultrasonic waves are transmitted through your thyroid and recorded by a scanning machine. The procedure is painless and does not use radioactive isotopes.

The thyroid ultrasound is useful for some patients with thyroid nodules who are difficult to examine because of large neck muscles. The results can then be used as a basis of comparison for any subsequent changes. Although thyroid size and the number and size of any nodules can be determined by ultrasound, the procedure gives no information regarding the presence of thyroid cancer. Thyroid ultrasound generally costs between $100 and $200.

Special Tests

Other tests that provide an image of your thyroid gland, such as computerized tomography (CT) or magnetic resonance imaging (MRI), are rarely necessary in the evaluation of a nodular goiter. Such tests are expensive, $300 to $500 for computerized tomography and $800 to $1,200 for magnetic resonance imaging. They usually provide little information that cannot be obtained by thyroid ultrasound, which is much less costly.

These special tests occasionally may be useful in the patient whose goiter is suspected of compressing the trachea, the esophagus, or the nerves that move the muscles supplying the vocal cords.

NODULAR GOITER AND CANCER OF THE THYROID

Having a nodular goiter does not put you at increased risk of thyroid cancer, unless one of the nodules is particularly hard and is "cold," or functioning poorly according to the radioactive iodide scan. Thyroid cancer, which is a rare disease compared to nodular goiter (see chapter 17), can develop over time in patients with nodular goiter, just as it can develop in those who do not have any detectable thyroid disease.

Since nodular goiters may occasionally obscure the presence of a small thyroid cancer, it is particularly important for you to schedule regular follow-up visits to your doctor so that any suspiciously enlarged, hard areas can be detected early.

A referral to an endocrinologist is often necessary to determine whether diagnostic tests to detect thyroid cancer, such as aspiration biopsy, are warranted (see chapter 17).

DEVELOPMENT OF HYPERTHYROIDISM

TSH Levels

Some nodular goiters cause hyperthyroidism, but most patients do not have hyperthyroidism when their nodular goiter is first discovered. You may, however, have a decrease in your serum TSH to less than 0.1 µU/ml, the earliest indication that your thyroid has begun to overproduce thyroid hormone. This places you at an increased risk for future development of hyperthyroid symptoms.

Some patients with nodular goiter have an enlarging mass of nodular tissue that overproduces thyroid hormone, eventually resulting in the symptoms and disability of hyperthyroidism (see chapter 6). Since a decrease in your serum TSH is the most sensitive indicator of developing hyperthyroidism, determination of your serum TSH is an essential part of your follow-up evaluation.

Excess Iodide

Many patients with nodular goiter will be at risk of developing hyperthyroidism if they are exposed to very large amounts of iodide. Exposure to excessive iodide often occurs during various X-ray diagnostic procedures such as intravenous pyelogram (IVP), which is used to visualize the kidneys and bladder; angiography, a test to visualize the blood vessels of the heart or other organs; and when contrast material is used in conjunction with CT scans.

X-ray contrast material contains large amounts of iodide, which can lead to hyperthyroidism when given to a patient with a nodular goiter. Therefore, if you have nodular goiter and you must have one of the X-ray diagnostic procedures requiring contrast material, your doctor should watch you closely for development of hyperthyroidism.

Treatment

Because of the differences in the rate of enlargement of the goiter, no single treatment is appropriate for all patients. If you are over 60 years of age with a small, recently discovered nodular goiter, your doctor may appropriately decide to observe the goiter over time without any specific treatment. You should be examined every three to six months for the first year and, if no changes occur in the size or consistency of your nodules, every 6 to 12 months thereafter. Such a goiter almost always remains innocuous and will not cause any medical problems.

However, if your goiter is discovered when you are young or middle-aged, its potential for growth will be uncertain. You should therefore be observed more closely and probably treated with L-thyroxine.

Treatment with L-Thyroxine

The goal of L-thyroxine treatment is first to decrease your serum TSH to less than 0.1 μU/ml and then to determine the effect of this therapy on the size of your goiter. Even though TSH is not directly responsible for the growth of many goiters, it may facilitate further growth. The general principles for administration of L-thyroxine are similar to those for L-thyroxine treatment of hypothyroidism (see chapter 13), and the dosage will be adjusted upward to the lowest dose that results in a decrease in your serum TSH. Such a TSH-suppressive dose of L-thyroxine should not produce symptoms or signs of hyperthyroidism in young or middle-aged patients.

The response to L-thyroxine treatment varies among different patients, depending to some extent on the characteristics of their goiter. If it is uniform or diffuse, without nodules, its size will probably decrease substantially during L-thyroxine treatment, and it may even disappear. You can then be maintained on L-thyroxine, which will continue to deprive your thyroid of the growth stimulation of TSH.

Treatment can be discontinued after one to three years to determine whether your thyroid will remain normal in size or whether the goiter will recur. In the latter case, you should probably be maintained on lifelong L-thyroxine treatment at a dosage that is demonstrated to maintain your serum TSH in the normal range or slightly below the normal range, but not decreased to less than 0.1 μU/ml.

Failure of L-Thyroxine Treatment

If you have a nodular goiter, the initial effect of L-thyroxine treatment on the size of your goiter will usually be much less significant than in diffuse goiter. Most treated patients have only a modest decrease in goiter size (perhaps 20 to 50 percent), and some may experience no change in size at all. The lack of a decrease or increase in the size of your goiter during L-thyroxine treatment indicates that treatment has been ineffective and that your nodular goiter may continue to be a medical problem for the rest of your life. Surgical removal of the goiter may then be appropriate for such patients.

The responses to L-thyroxine treatment fall between the extremes listed above, so that a specific therapeutic recommendation must take into account your wishes, particularly with respect to surgery, and your ability to live your life with annual medical follow-up.

16

THYROID NODULES

Few situations in life are more frightening than discovering a lump anywhere in your body, because of the immediate fear of a tumor or cancer. Although a lump or nodule in the thyroid gland may indeed be thyroid cancer, the risk of a malignancy is relatively low, only about 5 to 15 percent.

Any nodule must be evaluated by your doctor by means of medical history, physical examination, and special diagnostic tests. Most of the time, an accurate diagnosis can be made at relatively low cost and with little risk or discomfort. Only a minority of patients with thyroid nodules who are suspected of having thyroid cancer will be referred for surgery (see chapter 17). The majority will be treated with thyroid hormone by their internists or endocrinologists.

EVALUATING NODULES

Thyroid nodules are usually discovered by patients, their friends, or their doctors in much the same way as are goiters (see chapter 15). Your doctor will begin investigating the cause of your nodule with a careful medical history, since it will often provide important clues relating to the presence or absence of malignancy. Thyroid cancers tend to enlarge slowly over the course of time. Therefore, if your thyroid nodule has been present for years and has not changed significantly either in its size or consistency, it is almost certainly benign. Similarly, if your nodule appeared suddenly, almost overnight, it is likely to be a collection of fluid, or a cyst. Most thyroid cysts are benign. In addition, if you are found to have hyperthyroidism or Hashimoto's thyroiditis, the odds are that your nodule is benign.

RISK FACTORS

There are several risk factors for thyroid malignancy:

1. A nodule that continues to enlarge while you are being treated with L-thyroxine at a dosage that decreases serum TSH could be malignant. Since TSH is the most potent growth factor for thyroid tissue in your body, growth of your nodule in the absence of TSH strongly suggests thyroid cancer.

2. The risk of malignancy is greater if the nodule appears at a very young age or in a male older than 50 years of age.

3. You are at risk for thyroid cancer if you experience difficulty in swallowing food or liquids, if you wheeze, or if you have recently noticed hoarseness. These complaints frequently indicate spread of thyroid cancer outside of your thyroid gland, causing compression or invasion of your trachea, your esophagus, or one of the nerves that control your vocal cords.

4. Pain may be an indication of malignancy. The spread of thyroid cancer in the neck tissues may cause some pain or tenderness in the area of the nodule or up the side of your neck, and in your jawbone or ear.

5. If you underwent radiation therapy to your face, neck, or chest in early childhood, your risk for thyroid malignancy increases more than tenfold. If you subsequently develop a nodule, you must have it diagnosed as soon as possible. Radiation therapy, which was used before 1960 for enlarged tonsils or adenoids, various skin conditions, and a large thymus (an organ inside an infant's chest), is associated with the development of both benign and malignant thyroid nodules beginning about 15 years after the radiation. The risk continues throughout life.

PHYSICAL EXAMINATION

A careful physical examination is particularly important in the investigation of thyroid nodules. Once a nodule is discovered, usually by you or your family physician, you should be examined by either an internist or an endocrinologist who has experience treating patients with thyroid diseases.

Your doctor will determine how many nodules are present; whether their consistency is soft, normal, or hard in comparison to normal thyroid tissue; whether they remain suspiciously fixed in one position, or move up and down appropriately when you swallow; and whether lymph nodes adjacent to the nodule are enlarged. If your nodule is hard, does not move when you swallow, and is associated with one or more enlarged lymph nodes, you almost certainly have thyroid cancer. However, if your nodule is soft, moves normally, and is not associated with enlarged lymph nodes, you will likely have a benign nodule.

Based on the findings of the physical examination, your doctor will decide what laboratory tests and other procedures will be necessary for a determination of benign or malignant disease.

BLOOD TESTS

Although simple blood tests usually will not determine whether your thyroid nodule is benign or malignant, measurement of your serum T_4, TSH, and antithyroid microsomal antibodies still should be done when your nodule is discovered. A small increase in your serum T_4 and a decrease in your serum TSH to less than 0.1 μU/ml indicate that you have subclinical hyperthyroidism (see chapter 6) and strongly suggests that your thyroid nodule is functioning and therefore almost certainly benign (see chapter 10).

If these blood tests show a rise in your serum TSH and the presence of antithyroid microsomal antibodies, then you have subclinical hypothyroidism (see chapter 11) due to Hashimoto's thyroiditis (see chapter 12). Although the incidence of thyroid cancer is somewhat greater in persons with Hashimoto's disease than in those without thyroid disease, Hashimoto's thyroiditis is very common, whereas thyroid cancer is relatively rare. Therefore, if you have a thyroid nodule and are shown to have previously undiagnosed Hashimoto's thyroiditis, it is likely that your nodule is related to Hashimoto's and not due to thyroid cancer.

CALCITONIN MEASUREMENT

The only blood test that absolutely confirms that cancer is present within your thyroid gland is measurement of serum *calcitonin*, a hormone that affects the process of bone breakdown and reformation that continues throughout your life.

Certain thyroid tumors, known as *medullary* cancers of the thyroid (see chapter 17), always produce large amounts of calcitonin that can readily be measured in the blood serum. If your serum calcitonin concentration is increased, your thyroid nodule almost certainly contains medullary thyroid cancer, whereas a serum calcitonin concentration that is within the normal range indicates that your nodule is not a medullary thyroid cancer.

THYROID SCAN

A thyroid scan will indicate the function of your thyroid nodule. Functioning thyroid nodules, which account for about 10 to 20 percent of all thyroid nodules, have a very low incidence of thyroid cancer. Since they will trap radioactive iodide as well or better than normal thyroid tissue can, the finding that your nodule contains increased amounts of radioactivity compared to a nonnodular area means that your nodule has either normal or autonomous function (see chapter 10). It establishes that your thyroid nodule is benign, eliminating the need for any further testing.

Most thyroid nodules, about 80 percent, trap radioactive iodide poorly when compared to normal thyroid tissue. In such cases, the thyroid scan shows much less of the radioactive iodide localized in the area of your thyroid nodule (Figure 16.1). This finding, commonly called a *cold nodule*, means

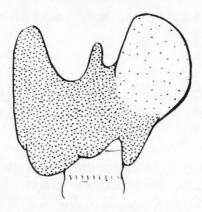

Figure 16.1 Radioactive iodide scan of a patient with a nonfunctioning ("cold") thyroid nodule. A nodule in the left lobe of the thyroid gland was felt by the doctor but found to contain little radioactive iodide. This is indicated above by fewer dots.

that your nodule has about a 10 to 20 percent chance of being thyroid cancer. If you have a cold nodule, only a biopsy will determine whether your nodule is benign or malignant.

THYROID ULTRASOUND

Many physicians routinely order a thyroid ultrasound test when they order a radioactive iodide scan, but ultrasound tests do *not* distinguish between benign nodules and thyroid cancer. The purpose of ultrasound testing is to determine whether your nodule is composed of solid tissue, possibly cancer, or a fluid-filled cyst that is usually associated with benign disease.

Since thyroid aspiration biopsy will easily show whether your nodule is a fluid-filled cyst, and since all patients who are discovered to have a "cold nodule" on thyroid scan will have a thyroid biopsy for accurate tissue diagnosis, the thyroid ultrasound is not necessary for the routine investigation of a thyroid nodule.

THYROID ASPIRATION BIOPSY

This is the single most important test for determining whether your thyroid nodule is benign or malignant. Before the technique and interpretation of this biopsy were perfected, most patients with a cold nodule on thyroid scan were referred directly for surgical removal of their nodule. Since thyroid cancer was found in only about 20 percent of these patients, four out of five patients were undergoing surgery just to determine that they did not have thyroid cancer.

Thyroid aspiration biopsy now provides a clear-cut diagnosis of benign or malignant disease in 60 to 70 percent of patients with a "cold nodule" on thyroid scan, allowing endocrinologists to carry out medical therapy for the majority of patients with benign disease. Using the aspiration biopsy as a guide for selecting patients, the incidence of thyroid cancer in patients referred for surgery is now about 50 to 60 percent, indicating that fewer patients with benign disease are now being sent to surgery to establish a diagnosis.

Procedure

You should not be apprehensive about having a thyroid aspiration biopsy. It is a safe procedure and does not cause much more discomfort than having a routine blood sample taken from one of the veins in your arm.

A fine needle, much thinner than the needle used for drawing samples of blood, is attached to a syringe and inserted directly into your thyroid nodule. Some doctors will numb your skin with novocaine or temporarily freeze it with an ethyl chloride spray, but these procedures may be more uncomfortable than the aspiration biopsy itself. The drop of fluid obtained from your nodule by suction on the syringe, which contains thyroid cells, is smeared on glass slides that are subsequently stained and examined by cytologists.

Complications from fine-needle aspiration biopsy of thyroid nodules are rare. Most patients experience no significant discomfort during the procedure; only a few develop slight tenderness over the area of the biopsy or a small black-and-blue mark at the puncture site.

DIAGNOSIS

Some diagnoses of benign or malignant thyroid disease are relatively easy to make from thyroid aspiration smears, but others are difficult because the findings are subtle. If there is any uncertainty concerning the diagnosis, the slides can always be reviewed by another cytologist. A second aspiration biopsy can also be done to obtain more tissue.

As noted above, aspiration biopsy usually results in a clear-cut diagnosis in about 60 percent of patients. Samples containing sufficient thyroid tissue for analysis are not obtained even on repeated biopsy in 15 to 20 percent of patients. In the remaining 20 percent, findings are either not diagnostic for either benign or malignant disease or show cells that are "suspicious" but not clearly tumor cells. This last group of patients and those with an established diagnosis of thyroid cancer will be referred for surgery.

SURGERY

Your surgeon will remove the lobe of your thyroid containing the nodule and then wait in the operating room until a pathologist has prepared and interpreted a "frozen section" of your nodular tissue. This analysis is relatively crude compared to the interpretation of the final pathological slides, which takes two to three days. Still, it is rapid and is usually precise enough for the surgeon to know whether or not your nodule is cancerous.

If your nodule is interpreted to be benign based on frozen section, your surgeon will close the incision and that will be the extent of your surgery. If your nodule is determined to be malignant, your surgeon will use his or her best judgment in conjunction with the opinion of your endocrinologist to determine the extent of surgery necessary to cure your cancer. He or she may then proceed to remove more of your thyroid tissue, including any lymph nodes that are affected, or may decide that taking out the thyroid lobe that contained the cancer is enough (see next chapter).

Patients generally return home three to seven days after surgery, depending on the extent of the operation. In skilled hands, the incidence of complications such as damage to the nerve supplying the vocal cords or damage to the parathyroid glands regulating your serum calcium should be low—about 1 to 3 percent—even if all of your thyroid tissue has been removed.

MEDICAL TREATMENT

Lifelong treatment with L-thyroxine is indicated in all patients who have had thyroid surgery for cancer or benign thyroid nodules. The dosage will vary depending on whether you had thyroid cancer or a benign disease.

If you had thyroid cancer, your dosage should be sufficient to decrease your serum TSH to less than 0.1 µU/ml (see chapter 17). If your surgery revealed a benign disease, your dosage of L-thyroxine should be sufficient to maintain serum TSH in the lower part of the normal range.

Guidelines for administration of L-thyroxine are similar to those for the treatment of hypothyroidism (see chapter 13). Follow-up examination should be carried out at yearly intervals and should include careful examination of your neck to detect any development of new nodules at the earliest time, as well as measurement of your serum T_4 and TSH.

If you did not have surgery because your aspiration biopsy revealed that your nodule was benign, you should still be treated with L-thyroxine, both to decrease the size of your nodule and to limit further growth. The initial dosage of L-thyroxine will be the minimal amount necessary to decrease your serum TSH to below the normal range, and this dose may be maintained for 6 to 12 months. The usual response to this treatment is a modest reduction in nodule size. Thereafter, the dosage should probably be decreased to one that maintains your serum TSH in the lower portion of the normal range. This will avoid potential long-term complications of subclinical hyperthyroidism, as well as a decrease in the mineral content of your bones and possible deleterious effects on your heart.

17

THYROID CANCER

Thyroid cancer is usually diagnosed by means of a fine-needle aspiration biopsy of a thyroid nodule (see chapter 16). In patients whose aspiration biopsy was either suspicious or ambiguous, thyroid tissue is surgically removed and evaluated. More than 90 percent of thyroid cancers arise from cells that originally manufactured and secreted thyroid hormones.

PAPILLARY AND FOLLICULAR CANCER

The two most frequent types of thyroid cancer have some features in common, and the treatment is similar. *Papillary* cancer contains tumor cells that form fingerlike, or papillary, structures; *follicular* cancer often contains follicles similar to those of normal thyroid tissue. When appropriate treatment begins at a relatively early stage, more than 90 percent of patients will be cured of these cancers.

Papillary cancers occur mainly in young to middle-aged individuals and tend to spread gradually throughout the thyroid gland, to the lymph nodes surrounding the thyroid gland, and eventually to other nearby structures such as the neck muscles, trachea, and esophagus. (Distant sites such as the lungs or bones are not usually affected until very late in the disease.)

In contrast, follicular thyroid cancer generally develops later in life, tends to invade the blood vessels and nerves within the thyroid gland at an early stage of the disease, and spreads to distant locations.

The best chance for cure of these cancers is early diagnosis and treatment begun when the tumors are still confined to the thyroid gland. Surgical treatment in conjunction with thyroid hormone therapy and radioactive iodide both for tumor detection and treatment should cure almost all patients whose cancers are still contained within the thyroid gland or localized to the neck. Effective treatment may be possible even when cancer has spread to sites distant from the thyroid, such as the lungs or bones.

Choosing a Surgeon

Because surgery is the primary therapy for thyroid cancer, your endocrinologist will refer you to a surgeon if your aspiration biopsy is positive, suspicious, or ambiguous for cancer. Since you will have the best chance for cure with the lowest complication rate if your surgeon has substantial experience treating thyroid cancer, you should be certain of your surgeon's qualifications and experience before scheduling surgery. Papillary and follicular thyroid cancers grow slowly, so you should not rush into an operation before you determine your doctor's credentials.

Surgeons trained primarily in surgery of the head and neck and some otorhinolaryngologists (ear, nose, and throat surgeons) are those who have the widest experience operating on thyroid cancer and, therefore, promise the best results. Their expertise will usually be widely recognized in their community. As their prospective patient, you should verify their medical reputations. In addition to checking their qualifications, ask your own doctor which surgeon has the best track record in the treatment of thyroid cancer.

Extent of Surgery

When you are referred for surgery, one of your first questions will probably be "How much of my thyroid will be removed?" Your surgeon's answer will be "As much as necessary to cure your cancer." Your surgeon will have to use his or her clinical judgment during the operation to decide how much of your thyroid tissue should be removed in order to cure your cancer.

If you have a small papillary thyroid cancer (less than 1.5 cm in diameter), most doctors will agree that a *lobectomy*—removal of only the lobe of your thyroid that contains the tumor—will cure you, and with almost no complications.

Similarly, most surgeons will agree that complete removal of the thyroid, called a *total thyroidectomy*, is the appropriate operation for a large papillary cancer (more than 3 cm in diameter) that invades both of your thyroid lobes.

The extent of surgery necessary to produce the best result for tumors that are intermediate in size is still debated by many surgeons. For example, there is still no consensus among surgeons about how much surgery should be done to cure a large papillary cancer that seems, on examination, to be confined to only one lobe. The same is true of a small follicular thyroid cancer that, on microscopic examination, seems to be invading blood vessels within your thyroid. Total thyroidectomy is probably the most appropriate operation for both tumors, but the experienced surgeon must make a judgment during the operation.

THE SURGICAL PROCEDURE

Necklace Incision

Removal of the thyroid is usually carried out through a "necklace" incision in the lower part of your neck. Many patients are surprised that the incision goes across the neck from side to side, rather than being a small incision directly over the thyroid tumor. Although the recommended incision is a wide one, it is actually safer for you because it allows your surgeon not only to completely remove your tumor but also to identify all of the important normal structures, including the parathyroid glands, and thereby avoid damaging them. A wider incision also gives your surgeon the opportunity to examine the remainder of your neck by probing with his or her fingers and examining the area visually, looking for enlargement of lymph nodes.

If your thyroid cancer has spread to several lymph nodes adjacent to your thyroid gland, they will be removed along with the gland. When an experienced surgeon carries out the procedure, the cure rate for papillary thyroid cancer that has spread to several adjacent lymph nodes is just as high as when the tumor is confined to the gland itself.

Radical Neck Dissection

If numerous enlarged lymph nodes are discovered in your neck either before or during surgery, and they cannot be completely removed through the original necklace incision, your surgeon may decide to perform a radical neck dissection rather than a thyroidectomy, looking for enlarged lymph nodes invaded by a tumor.

In a neck dissection, the necklace incision is extended upwards on one side of the neck to behind the ear. All tissue from the upper neck to the lower neck, including the lymph nodes and the thyroid gland, is then removed in one piece. Left intact are the carotid artery and jugular vein, the principal blood vessels supplying the head and brain; several critical nerves; and the neck muscles, if they appear free of tumor.

In contrast to a thyroidectomy, which leaves only a necklace scar as permanent evidence of your surgery, a radical neck dissection leaves a more extensive scar. Depending on the amount of muscle tissue removed, there will be some hollowing of the front of your neck. Neck dissection should be done only by an expert, and only as a curative procedure.

Maintaining Normal Thyroid Function

Some patients are concerned that they will suffer serious disability once their thyroid gland has been completely removed, but this is not the case. Tablets containing synthetic L-thyroxine that is identical to the thyroid hormone previously secreted by your thyroid gland will maintain normal thyroid function (see chapter 13).

Damage to the Vocal Cords and the Parathyroids

Of greater concern are two complications that may occur after thyroid surgery: damage to the recurrent laryngeal nerve, one of the nerves that controls your vocal cords, and damage to the parathyroid glands.

In experienced surgical hands, damage to this nerve should occur in less than 1 percent of patients, so long as the tumor has not directly invaded the area of the nerve. However, in some patients whose tumor involves the recurrent laryngeal nerve, the nerve may have to be removed in order to better the chance for cure of the thyroid cancer. Permanent hoarseness results from damage or removal of the nerve.

The four tiny parathyroid glands are located in pairs on either side of the neck, just behind the thyroid gland. They secrete a protein called parathyroid hormone, or PTH, which is essential for maintaining a normal concentration of calcium in your blood serum. Since normal function of even one of these four glands is sufficient to produce a normal amount of parathyroid hormone, it takes severe damage to all of these glands to cause a deficiency in PTH secretion and a consequent decrease in serum calcium. Normal parathyroid glands are often difficult to locate even by the most experienced surgeons, and all four glands may be inadvertently damaged in 1 to 3 percent of patients undergoing total thyroidectomy.

Calcium Deficiency

For the first several days after neck surgery, your serum calcium will be measured at least twice each day. A small decline in serum calcium, causing some tingling around your lips and in your fingers, may occur after surgery and can be treated for several days with oral or intravenous calcium.

Permanent damage to your parathyroid glands, leading to chronic and severe deficiency in your blood calcium (hypoparathyroidism), can be treated very satisfactorily with large doses of vitamin D or a small amount of an active form of vitamin D, called Rocaltrol, together with supplemental calcium. Like thyroid hormone treatment, once a dosage of vitamin D and calcium is established for you, you should see your doctor every three to six months for examination and measurement of serum calcium to determine whether the dosage needs adjustment.

MANAGEMENT AFTER SURGERY

Radioactive Iodide Scanning

After surgery, a scan using radioactive iodide will enable your endocrinologist to detect any remaining thyroid tissue or tumor tissue. If those tissues are found, they must be destroyed with an additional dose of radioactive iodide.

There are several differences in the use of radioactive iodide for diagnostic scanning (see chapters 5 and 10) and for the detection of tumor deposits, called *metastases*.

First, a different form (isotope) of radioactive iodide will be used for cancer detection, a form that produces more energy, enabling it to penetrate the tissues, exit the body, and be detected by appropriate scanning machines. A small deposit of thyroid cancer that accumulates radioactive iodide may thereby be detected; it would not be detected with the isotope used for routine scanning of goiters or nodules.

A second difference is that your endocrinologist will use a high scanning dose of radioactive iodide (2–10 millicuries) when screening for tumors, rather than the very small doses (0.1–0.3 millicuries) that are used to determine the function of thyroid nodules (see chapter 16).

Scanning with radioactive iodide will be delayed for four to six weeks after your surgery in order to ensure complete healing of all of the tissues in your neck. In the time between your surgery and your first radioactive iodide scan, your endocrinologist will prescribe a small dosage of thyroid hormone to prevent you from developing the full-blown symptoms and signs of hypothyroidism (see chapter 11). Your thyroid hormone treatment will be stopped 10 days to two weeks before the radioactive iodide scan in order to allow serum TSH levels to rise. Radioactive iodide testing for the presence of small tumor deposits is much more sensitive when your serum TSH is significantly increased, with the result that, unfortunately, you will experience some symptoms of hypo-thyroidism (see chapter 11). This scanning procedure should be simplified within the next few years, because injectible human TSH has just become available for use in humans. Initial studies indicate that it is safe and, when injected into patients who are still taking their thyroid hormone medication, detects small tumor deposits in the same way as the original procedure. Using this new human TSH, patients will not have to stop taking their medication and suffer symptoms of hypo-thyroidism while waiting to have their radioactive iodide scans.

If the scan reveals a small amount of residual normal thyroid tissue, your endocrinologist or nuclear medicine physician will administer a dose of radioactive iodide large enough to destroy it.

Even though thyroid cancers appear "cold" (do not accumulate radioactive iodide) on a radioactive iodide scan compared to your normal thyroid (see chapter 16), more than half of them actually do accumulate radioactive iodide, but at a rate that is about 1 percent of the total amount taken by normal thyroid tissue. If all of your normal thyroid tissue is surgically removed or destroyed with radioactive iodide, even this low rate of radioactive iodide accumulation by tumor tissue will frequently be sufficient to visualize the abnormal tissue with a scan.

Radioactive Iodide Treatment

A treatment dose of radioactive iodide for destruction of a small remnant of normal thyroid tissue is generally in the range of 30 to 100 millicuries. In some treatment centers, the entire amount is given in one dose during a hospitalization of several days. Since Nuclear Regulatory Commission regulations require that you be hospitalized for doses in excess of 30 millicuries of iodide, many centers will administer one or more doses of 30 millicuries of iodide to you as an outpatient. As in radioactive iodide therapy for hyperthyroidism (see chapter 8), radioactive iodide that is not accumulated by your thyroid tissue remnants will be excreted in your urine. Careful toilet-flushing and handwashing will prevent contamination. Radioactive iodide will also appear in your saliva (see chapter 8).

You should not fear receiving treatment doses of radioactive iodide, because you will not feel any different after you take it. It is generally given in capsules that are tasteless. Drinking a few extra 8-ounce glasses of water each day for the first several days after radioactive iodide treatment will increase your frequency of urination, facilitating excretion of the radioactive iodide that is not accumulated by thyroid tissue and lessening the exposure of other tissues in your body to radiation. Detailed instructions concerning exposure of other individuals will vary according to the dosage of radioactive iodide and will be given to you by your endocrinologist or nuclear medicine physician.

Thyroid Hormone Treatment

The best results in the care of patients with thyroid cancer are obtained when initial surgery has removed all tumor tissue or when subsequent treatment with radioactive iodide has destroyed remaining tumor deposits. This occurs in about 90 percent of patients with papillary cancer and in perhaps 50 to 75 percent of patients with follicular cancer. Since your doctor can never be absolutely sure that you are completely tumor-free, the goal of long-term treatment is to keep you feeling well and functioning normally, to detect any residual tumor at the earliest possible time, and to eliminate the tumor either by surgery or by using radioactive iodide.

Thyroid hormone treatment, a mainstay in the long-term

management of thyroid cancer, is administered for two reasons: (1) to prevent the severe hypothyroidism that would develop following removal of all your thyroid tissue, and (2) to maintain your serum TSH at very low levels, because serum TSH is a potent growth stimulator for thyroid tissue, including many thyroid cancers. The general guidelines for thyroid hormone treatment are similar to those for treatment of hypothyroidism (see chapter 13), but the dosage will be adjusted upward to the minimal dose that causes a decrease in your serum TSH to less than 0.1 μU/ml.

Long-Term Management

Even though you will be feeling well, you should still see your endocrinologist every three to six months for the first year or two after surgery for thyroid cancer. Your doctor will carefully examine your neck to detect residual tumor or enlarged lymph nodes and will also measure your serum TSH to ensure that your dosage of L-thyroxine is sufficient to suppress TSH.

An additional important blood test is measurement of serum thyroglobulin, a protein that is unique to thyroid tissue (see chapter 1). Since all of your thyroid gland was removed, you should have virtually no thyroglobulin in your blood. The presence of normal or raised concentrations of serum thyroglobulin indicates that you have residual thyroid cancer, which can then be located by radioactive iodide scanning, chest X-ray, or CT scan.

Recurrent Cancer

A recurrence of your cancer should be removed surgically or destroyed with radioactive iodide. External radiation therapy, used for treatment of many other types of cancer, and chemotherapy are generally ineffective.

A recurrent tumor that seems localized to the neck will

probably be removed surgically because surgical exploration may identify other tumor deposits not detected by physical examination, CT scan, or even radioactive iodide scans.

If thyroid cancer metastases occur at distant sites, for example in your lungs or bones, radioactive iodide is the treatment of choice. Large doses—between 100 and 200 millicuries—must be given during a hospital stay. Such doses may be associated with swelling and discomfort of your salivary glands, lasting for one or two days. Another common complaint is minor stomach upset, but most patients experience no particular discomfort at all.

Cure

A cure rate of 95 percent for papillary cancer and 80 to 95 percent for follicular cancer is common for cancer restricted to the neck. If your neck examination, radioactive iodide scan, and chest X ray remain negative and your serum thyroglobulin concentration remains undetectable for five years after surgery, you can consider yourself cured. Only rarely does a tumor recur after five years of quiescence. However, you should still be examined at annual intervals, and the evaluation should include measurement of your serum TSH and thyroglobulin.

MEDULLARY CANCER

Medullary cancers arise from nonthyroid cells within the thyroid gland that produce large amounts of a protein called calcitonin, not thyroid hormones (see chapter 16). Since the cells of this cancer are not of thyroid origin, they do not concentrate radioactive iodide, secrete thyroid hormones or thyroglobulin, and do not respond to suppression of serum TSH.

The best management of these cancers seems to be aggressive surgical removal, often with radical neck dissection if the tumor has already spread to local lymph nodes in the neck.

Follow-up management includes thyroid hormone treatment that maintains you in the euthyroid state (see chapter 13) but does not suppress your serum TSH. Another necessary measurement is serum calcitonin concentration. Undetectable or low serum calcitonin concentrations over several years usually indicate a cure. However, an increased concentration of serum calcitonin or a rising serum calcitonin concentration indicates the presence of residual medullary cancer, which will be identified by appropriate X ray, CT, or MRI scanning. Residual tumor should be removed surgically, if it can be done safely, or else treated with external radiation therapy. Chemotherapy is generally not successful.

The course of medullary cancer of the thyroid is quite variable and, therefore, the outcome is unpredictable. Some patients seem to have very aggressive tumors that will be fatal within three to five years, whereas others, even with significantly increased serum calcitonin concentration indicating residual tumor, may live for many years without progression of the tumor or any apparent disability.

Occasionally, medullary carcinoma of the thyroid may be a familial disease associated with hypertension. All patients with medullary carcinoma should be evaluated by an endocrinologist to determine if their disease has the characteristics of the familial form. If so, blood relatives should be examined and tested—using serum calcitonin measurements—to detect the presence of a tumor. Affected family members can now be identified through serum calcitonin measurements and genetic markers and their thyroid glands can be removed even before cancer develops.

ANAPLASTIC CANCER

This is an uncommon type of thyroid cancer, accounting for less than 5 percent of all thyroid cancers. Unresponsive to all currently available treatments, anaplastic cancer generally leads to death within one year. It is usually discovered as a hard, irregular mass in the thyroid, with adjacent enlarged and hard lymph nodes.

After needle aspiration biopsy confirms the diagnosis, attempts at surgical removal are questionable because such patients are never cured by surgery. The disease does not respond to lowering of serum TSH with thyroid hormone therapy or to radioactive iodide, but it may respond for a limited period of time to external radiation therapy or to chemotherapy. Patients with anaplastic cancer of the thyroid should therefore be referred for supportive treatment to a radiation therapist or oncologist.

18

THYROID DISEASE AND PREGNANCY

Since thyroid disease is most prevalent in women of child-bearing age, it is not surprising that many women ask how their thyroid problem will affect a current or future pregnancy and if the treatment itself will harm their unborn children. Thyroid dysfunction can alter your fertility, the outcome of your pregnancy, and the health of your baby; it also may appear as a consequence of your pregnancy.

HYPOTHYROIDISM

Effects on Fertility

If you have severe hypothyroidism, you will likely have irregular and heavy menstrual flow, as well as flow between your periods (see chapter 11). Most women with hypothyroidism do not ovulate regularly, which significantly decreases their fertility. In fact, your hypothyroidism may be diagnosed for the first time when you have a medical evaluation for infertility. If you have a milder degree of hypothyroidism, especially subclinical hypothyroidism (see chapter 12), you may have normal fertility, but the outcome of your pregnancy may still be compromised.

Miscarriage and Other Risks

When you are hypothyroid, the odds that you will have a miscarriage are doubled and, if you carry your baby into the eighth or ninth month, your risks are also increased for developing high blood pressure and possibly kidney damage, for having an abrupt delivery with excessive bleeding, or other complications.

In the unusual circumstance that you are able both to conceive and to carry your child to term despite severe hypothyroidism, your newborn will be at increased risk for impaired mental and physical development.

Importance of Early Diagnosis and Treatment

Because of the very significant impact of hypothyroidism on pregnancy, you should under ideal circumstances be in good health before beginning your pregnancy or, if symptoms suggesting hypothyroidism develop at any time during your pregnancy (see chapter 11), you should see your doctor quickly for diagnosis and treatment.

Your doctor will carry out a careful history and physical examination and order measurements of your serum free T_4 and TSH concentrations. Free T_4 is the proper test because the large amounts of estrogens produced during your pregnancy will result in a rise in the serum-binding proteins for thyroid hormones (see chapter 5). If you have hypothyroidism due to thyroid gland disease, your serum-free T_4 should be decreased and the concentration of your serum TSH should be raised. Once hypothyroidism is diagnosed, it should be treated rapidly with L-thyroxine (see chapter 13).

Pregnancy and L-Thyroxine Treatment

Many hypothyroid patients who are already being treated with L-thyroxine ask whether their medication is safe during pregnancy.

In the dosage that is correct for you, L-thyroxine is not only safe for you and your developing baby but also essential; without it, you will again develop hypothyroidism, with all of its attendant harmful effects on pregnancy. Therefore, you should continue to take your L-thyroxine tablets when you are planning a pregnancy or find out that you are pregnant.

Moreover, if your serum thyroid hormone concentrations have not been measured during the last six months, you should see your doctor to determine whether your current dosage of L-thyroxine is still appropriate for you. Because some women require a modest increase in the dosage of L-thyroxine during pregnancy, your thyroid function should be evaluated in the second to third month and again in the sixth month of pregnancy. Your dosage of L-thyroxine can then be adjusted, if necessary. Once you have delivered, you can usually return to your previous dose of L-thyroxine, but this should be done under your doctor's supervision.

HYPERTHYROIDISM

Treatment Choices Before Pregnancy

If you are hyperthyroid, your plans for subsequent pregnancies are an important consideration in choosing between radioactive iodide treatment or management with propyl-thiouracil (PTU) or methimazole (see chapter 8).

Many patients develop hypothyroidism following radio-active iodide treatment, requiring therapy with L-thyroxine, and most patients treated with the antithyroid drugs PTU or methimazole do not enter remission. Therefore, you should anticipate the likelihood that you will be treated either with L-thyroxine or one of the antithyroid drugs during a future pregnancy.

L-thyroxine and antithyroid drugs. Since L-thyroxine is identical to your own thyroid hormone, it is perfectly safe both for you and your developing baby, as long as the dose is appropriately adjusted during pregnancy (see above).

Similarly, the antithyroid drugs are also safe when they are used in small doses—less than 20 mg per day for methimazole and less than 200 mg per day for PTU. Even though these antithyroid drugs do cross the placental barrier and enter the developing fetus's circulation, newborns of mothers treated with small doses of these drugs seem quite normal at birth and continue to develop normally.

However, if you have severe hyperthyroidism and require large daily doses of methimazole (more than 20 mg per day) or PTU (more than 200 mg per day), the medications may significantly inhibit your baby's thyroid function, causing thyroid enlargement and hypothyroidism. An alternative to large doses of antithyroid drugs for the control of hyperthyroidism in pregnancy is subtotal thyroidectomy, which is most safely carried out during the fourth through the sixth month of pregnancy.

Radioactive iodide treatment. If your hyperthyroidism is severe, requiring a large daily dose of PTU or methimazole to maintain you in a euthyroid state, it is safer in your subsequent pregnancies to have radioactive iodide treatment for your hyperthyroidism, even if you develop hypothyroidism and require daily L-thyroxine.

Plans for pregnancy should be delayed for 6 to 12 months after radioactive iodide treatment, not because of harmful effects of radioactive iodide on you or your future children but because thyroid function responds slowly to this treatment (see chapter 8). It may take three to six months of observation after therapy to determine whether you require a second dose of radioactive iodide to restore you to a euthyroid state.

Studies have shown that women treated with radioactive iodide before becoming pregnant have normal pregnancies. In addition, their babies' growth, development, and chance of having a congenital abnormality are no different than those of babies whose mothers had not taken radioactive iodide.

Hyperthyroidism During Pregnancy

Many women with normal pregnancies experience symptoms that are similar to those of hyperthyroidism. Because of a normal increase in the metabolic rate (see chapter 3) and the marked hormonal changes that occur during pregnancy, you may feel unusually warm or uncomfortable in warm environments. You may also notice that your heart rate is faster than normal even at rest, that you perspire excessively, and that your moods may swing widely during the ordinary stresses of daily life. If these symptoms are exaggerated, your doctor may suspect that you have mild hyperthyroidism in addition to your pregnancy.

Diagnosis. Your serum-free T_4 and TSH should be measured to determine whether your symptoms result from your pregnancy, which is most likely, or whether you also have mild hyperthyroidism. Results of both of these measurements are normal during pregnancy, but if you are hyperthyroid, your serum-free T_4 concentration will be raised and your serum TSH will be decreased to less than 0.1 μU/ml.

Treatment. If you have hyperthyroidism, you should be treated, because hyperthyroidism during pregnancy significantly increases your risk for a miscarriage. *Treatment with radioactive iodide is absolutely contraindicated* if you are pregnant or nursing, however. The radioactivity may affect the development of your baby and destroy the baby's thyroid.

Since hyperthyroidism that develops during pregnancy is generally mild, you will likely be treated with PTU in doses less than 200 mg per day. This drug enters your baby's circulation to a lesser extent than does methimazole.

If your hyperthyroidism is severe and not well controlled with a small dose of PTU, surgical removal of your thyroid is the next best choice for treatment, as radioactive iodide cannot be used. When carried out during the fourth through sixth months of pregnancy, surgery can generally be done successfully and without significantly increasing your risk of a miscarriage.

Hyperthyroidism and Your Newborn

Both the thyroid-stimulating antibodies that cause hyperthyroidism of Graves' disease (see chapter 7) and some of the drugs used to treat your hyperthyroidism may affect your newborn baby. Because the mother's antibodies always enter the baby's circulation near the end of pregnancy, high concentrations of thyroid-stimulating antibodies may result in hyperthyroidism in your newborn, persisting for several weeks or several months.

Since hyperthyroidism in your newborn is self-limited, your baby can simply be treated for several weeks with beta-blocking medications that reduce the effect of the adrenaline-like hormones (see chapter 8).

Your doctors should know that you have Graves' disease, and your pediatrician will observe your newborn closely for the presence of Graves'. You may still have thyroid-stimulating antibodies in your circulation even though you had Graves' disease that was treated with radioactive iodide before your current pregnancy.

Nursing. Many new mothers being treated for thyroid disease who intend to nurse their babies ask about the safety of L-thyroxine and the antithyroid drugs during nursing.

L-thyroxine does not appear in your breast milk and will not influence your baby. If you are hyperthyroid and are being treated either with PTU or methimazole, consult with your pediatrician and endocrinologist. These drugs will appear in your breast milk and, in high doses, may affect your baby's thyroid function. Most women who are taking small doses of PTU (less than 200 mg per day) or methimazole (less than 20 mg per day) can continue to take their medication and safely nurse their babies. However, the baby's thyroid function should be determined every two or three months.

THYROID PROBLEMS AFTER DELIVERY

The first months after your baby is born are often especially stressful, particularly if the baby is your first child. Recovery from the delivery itself and rapid and large changes in estrogen levels after delivery are quickly followed by the demands of caring for your newborn. Aside from fatigue and sleepless nights, some mothers who are nervous about the care of their new baby may develop symptoms of anxiety such as rapid heartbeat, excessive perspiration, and feelings of apprehension. Others may become somewhat lethargic and depressed. When these symptoms are mild, they interfere little with the care of your newborn and your other daily activities; when severe, however, as in postpartum depression, they may be disabling.

Hyperthyroidism

From recent reports in the medical literature, it is now clear that some of these complaints may be caused by thyroid dysfunction that commonly occurs during the first year after delivery. The second half of pregnancy is a time when many immune functions are decreased, including a rise in the antibodies that cause the hyperthyroidism of Graves' disease and the hypothyroidism of Hashimoto's thyroiditis. The concentration of these antibodies and their effects may increase rapidly after delivery.

If you have mild, even unsuspected, subclinical hyperthyroidism (see chapters 8 and 10) during pregnancy, it may worsen rapidly one or two months after delivery, causing symptoms of overactive thyroid (see chapter 6). If you experience palpitations, excessive perspiration, and nervousness after delivery, you should see your doctor and be evaluated by blood tests for an overactive thyroid (see chapter 5).

Graves' hyperthyroidism that appears after delivery will be treated the same way as hyperthyroidism in Graves' disease that is not associated with pregnancy or delivery, with one exception. If you are nursing your baby, radioactive iodide cannot be used because it will be concentrated in your breast milk as well as your thyroid, and thereby affect your baby. Also, if antithyroid drugs are used, the doses of these drugs should be low (see above).

Thyroiditis

More common than Graves' disease after delivery is the occurrence or worsening of thyroiditis of the Hashimoto's type, also known as postpartum thyroiditis. Evidence of thyroiditis can be detected in about 10 percent of women after delivery, making it a very common disorder. Some of the symptoms that develop after delivery, which are usually thought to be an exaggeration of expected changes, may well be due to postpartum thyroiditis.

If you develop postpartum thyroiditis, your symptoms will be similar to those of patients with silent thyroiditis (see chapter 14). You will first experience symptoms of an overactive thyroid (see chapter 6) and then develop symptoms of an underactive thyroid (see chapter 11). The hyperthyroid phase of your illness will occur within the first six months after delivery and may last for one to three months before it spontaneously resolves. You may then develop symptoms and signs of hypothyroidism, which will also resolve spontaneously after several weeks to several months.

Most women do not experience both the hyperthyroid and hypothyroid phases of the illnesses. Some have only one or the other. Evidence that disease exists may be determined on the basis of decreased or increased concentrations of serum T_4 and TSH.

The hyperthyroid phase. The hyperthyroid phase of postpartum thyroiditis can be diagnosed easily by finding an increase in your serum T_4 and a decrease in your serum TSH to less than 0.1 μU/ml. Your doctor will usually feel an enlargement of your thyroid gland, which is firm due to infiltration of lymphocytes. Antithyroid antibodies are usually increased in the blood. The uptake of radioactive iodide by your thyroid is the most reliable test to distinguish the hyperthyroidism of postpartum thyroiditis from that of Graves' disease. In

Graves' disease, the 24-hour radioactive iodide uptake will be increased above the normal range, whereas in hyperthyroidism of postpartum thyroiditis, the thyroidal uptake of radioactive iodide is decreased to less than 5 percent. Since the hyperthyroid phase is self-limited, lasting only one to two months, treatment is generally restricted to use of beta-blockers such as propranolol, which will relieve your symptoms. If your symptoms are relatively mild, you may not require any treatment at all.

The hypothyroid phase. The hypothyroid phase of postpartum thyroiditis generally occurs between 4 and 12 months after delivery and follows the hyperthyroid phase. It too is self-limited. Treatment with thyroid hormones should be given only for relief of symptoms of hypothyroidism, and should then be limited to several months, when you will be reevaluated.

Although long-term treatment for hypothyroidism should not be given on the basis of a single episode of postpartum thyroiditis, L-thyroxine treatment may be necessary later in life. If you have one or more episodes of postpartum thyroid dysfunction, you have a 20 to 30 percent chance of developing permanent hypothyroidism within five to ten years, which will require treatment. Therefore, you should certainly continue to be evaluated once a year for any evidence of thyroid malfunction.

19

THYROID DISEASE IN CHILDREN

CRETINISM

One of the great triumphs of modern endocrinology is the ability to eradicate *cretinism*, a centuries-old disorder resulting from hypothyroidism.

Because normal concentrations of thyroid hormones are essential both for development of the brain and for normal growth, babies who are hypothyroid at birth and remain untreated will have subnormal intelligence and will show poor physical development. Fortunately, most babies born with hypothyroidism but treated with L-thyroxine before three months of age will achieve normal intelligence.

Since effective treatment of hypothyroidism with thyroid hormone preparations has been available for nearly 100 years, only a failure to diagnose the disease in infants has resulted in children who are extremely short for their age and bloated with fluid, and who demonstrate below-normal intelligence.

Methods to measure thyroid hormones in blood, which were developed about 20 years ago, have now been added to neonatal screening programs for various congenital diseases. Today, all newborns—at least those who live in developed countries—are screened for hypothyroidism before they leave the hospital. Results of the hormone measurements are available within several days.

Congenital Screening Programs

Results of these screening programs indicate that the incidence of hypothyroidism at birth is about one in 4,000, making hypothyroidism one of the most common of the congenital disorders. Phenylketonuria (PKU), for example, has an incidence of about one in 30,000 births. Babies with hypothyroidism who are not diagnosed and treated at birth share certain characteristics: inactivity, feeding problems, constipation, large tongues, puffy facial features, and a bulge or hernia around the belly button. Over time, failure to grow and decreased intelligence will also become apparent.

As a result of congenital screening programs, appropriate diagnosis and treatment in the first weeks of life are not only possible but have now become standard practice in all developed countries. Treatment with thyroid hormone leads to normal growth and development as well as a normal IQ in over 90 percent of affected children. By means of congenital screening programs, it is now possible to eradicate congenital hypothyroidism and cretinism from the earth, a goal currently not realized in many countries because of economic, social, and political constraints.

Hypothyroidism

As in adults, the symptoms of hypothyroidism in children and adolescents may be variable and subtle, often leading to disability before the disorder is recognized.

Symptoms

The most characteristic feature of the disease is failure to grow (Figure 19.1). Therefore, your pediatrician's records of your child's growth will show slowing of growth to below the normal rate for your child's age. If your child falls off the normal curve because of slowed growth, hypothyroidism should be considered as the cause. Symptoms of hypothyroidism that occur in adults—constipation and dry skin—are not prominent in children. However, a delay in sexual development commonly occurs in older children, related in degree to the slowing of growth. If your child's growth is minimally af-

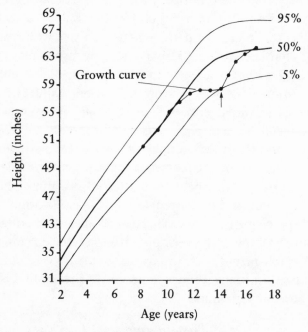

Figure 19.1. Hypothyroidism in children
This child was growing normally until growth slowed at age 11, when hypothyroidism developed. The child's growth rate was restored to normal after treatment with thyroid hormones, as indicated by the arrow.

fected by hypothyroidism, then puberty may progress normally. However, if your child's growth rate is severely impeded, the onset of puberty may also be substantially delayed.

Diagnosis

Once the possibility of hypothyroidism is considered by your doctor, the diagnosis is readily established by measurement of thyroid hormones and TSH. As in adults, a decrease in serum T_4 and a raised level of serum TSH in children indicate hypothyroidism and that the disorder is due to a disease of the thyroid gland.

The most common cause of thyroid disease in children is Hashimoto's thyroiditis (see chapter 12), and this is often associated with a high prevalence of Hashimoto's and Graves' disease in the adult members of the family, particularly in the women. Less frequently, growth failure and hypothyroidism during childhood or adolescence may also be the first indication of a pituitary or hypothalamic disease that may include other glandular deficiencies as well. The diagnosis of such problems and their treatment are similar to those of adult patients (see chapters 12 and 13).

Treatment

Treatment of hypothyroidism due to thyroid failure with L-thyroxine is similar to that of adults (see chapter 13). The goal of treatment is to normalize your child's serum T_4 and TSH and also to normalize the growth rate. Most children who are adequately treated will attain their expected adult height as long as their hypothyroidism was of reasonably short duration before treatment was started. If, however, the hypothyroidism was severe and prolonged (more than three years in duration), your child may not attain his or her predicted adult height.

Hyperthyroidism

Graves' disease is the most common cause of hyperthyroidism in children, usually occurring after five years of age, and with the greatest incidence in adolescence.

Symptoms

Children differ from adults in that their hyperthyroidism causes more emotional and behavioral problems and fewer physical symptoms (weight loss and excessive perspiration). When a child develops hyperthyroidism, a parent will usually take him or her to the doctor because of an increase in nervousness, wide swings in emotional behavior, and a decrease in the ability to concentrate, which often leads to a rapid decline in performance at school. Although hyperthyroid children show increased appetite, they do not experience the weight loss and increased frequency of bowel movements common in adults. Cardiac symptoms, particularly atrial fibrillation, occur infrequently in childhood hyperthyroidism.

On examination, the physician may note that your child's hands shake and that bulging eyes and muscle weakness are present. Usually, however, these conditions are not as severe as those seen in adult patients. Thyroid enlargement is usually present, but a child's goiter will not become large enough to cause symptoms of pressure in the front of the neck or difficulty swallowing food.

Diagnosis

A diagnosis of hyperthyroidism is established by finding that the child's serum T_4 is raised and that the serum TSH is decreased to less than 0.1 μU/ml. Since almost all children with hyperthyroidism have Graves' disease, a thyroid radioactive iodide uptake and scan are not indicated unless the thyroid contains a nodule. In that situation, a radioactive iodide scan should be done to determine whether the nodule accumulates ("warm") or doesn't accumulate radioactive iodide ("cold"). If it's "warm," it will certainly be a benign nodule. On the other hand, if it's "cold," it will have a 10 to 20 percent chance of being malignant (see chapter 16). Antithyroid antibodies will also be present, and the child will likely have adult family members who have had either Graves' disease or Hashimoto's thyroiditis. Thyroid-stimulating immunoglobulin, the cause of the hyperthyroidism (see chapter 8), can always be detected in children with hyperthyroidism, but it is rarely necessary to carry out this expensive measurement to diagnose hyperthyroidism or determine its cause.

Treatment

The available treatments for Graves' disease in adults—antithyroid drugs, radioactive iodide therapy, and surgery—are also employed in children with hyperthyroidism, but antithyroid drug treatment is preferred by most physicians more than is the use of radioactive iodide. The methods for using these treatments and the results of treatment are also similar to those observed in adults (see chapter 8).

Antithyroid drugs are employed in children because of lingering concern about long-term adverse effects after radioactive iodine treatment. Available research indicates that treatment of hyperthyroid adolescents with radioactive iodide is not associated with an increase in risk for thyroid cancer, leukemia, or congenital malformations in their offspring. The follow-up period for these studies is currently about 30 years, not the 60 to 75 years of life expectancy for these patients.

Therefore, many doctors attempt long-term treatment with one of the antithyroid drugs—methimazole or PTU—until either a remission occurs (see chapter 7) or the patient reaches young adulthood and can be treated with radioactive iodide.

When hyperthyroidism occurs in children, antithyroid drug treatment is often followed by surgical thyroidectomy. Surgery is indicated if remission does not occur or if the child becomes allergic to the medications.

20

THYROID DISEASE IN OLDER PEOPLE

HYPOTHYROIDISM

Diagnosing thyroid dysfunction in patients older than 65 is complicated by the fact that many of the symptoms of hypothyroidism are similar to those of the normal aging process.

Although some older people remain vigorous, most are aware of the gradual development of fatigue, declining muscle strength, increasing discomfort in cold environments, constipation, dry skin, and slowing of their thought processes.

The idea that some of the changes attributed to the normal aging process might be caused by thyroid hormone deficiency is not a new one. It was first suggested when it was found that the metabolic rate (see chapter 3) declines during aging, as it does in hypothyroidism.

Despite this coincidence of symptoms, measurements of thyroid hormones and TSH usually remain perfectly normal in later years, indicating that hypothyroidism is not responsible for the progressive symptoms of aging in the vast majority of patients.

Symptoms

Only 1 or 2 percent of older patients have a decrease in serum thyroid hormone concentrations and a rise in their serum TSH, indicating hypothyroidism. These patients may have marked symptoms suggesting hypothyroidism, similar to younger patients (see chapter 11), or their symptoms may be indistinguishable from the changes seen in normal aging. Those symptoms that are due to hypothyroidism will be relieved by treatment with thyroid hormones; those due to normal aging will not be affected by treatment.

However, up to 10 percent of older individuals, women more than men, have a significant increase in their serum TSH without a decrease in their serum thyroid hormone concentrations. This would suggest that they may have subclinical hypothyroidism (see chapter 13). At the present time, research has not yet determined whether these patients have more severe symptoms of normal aging or hypothyroidism than comparably aged patients with normal serum TSH. It is also uncertain whether treatment with thyroid hormones will reverse some or all of their complaints.

Diagnosis

Because of the difficulty in distinguishing between the presence of hypothyroidism and the normal aging process by means of a patient's history and physical examination, hypothyroidism in the older age group frequently remains undiagnosed. Many physicians will not suspect hypothyroidism when they receive complaints of fatigue, dry skin, and constipation.

Measurement of serum T_4 and TSH should therefore be done routinely in older patients, as part of their general medical evaluation. Older patients often ask their doctors about their blood sugar and cholesterol levels. They should also ask about their thyroid hormone blood levels.

Treatment Guidelines

Once a diagnosis is made, hypothyroidism is treated with L-thyroxine (see chapter 13), but the daily dosage is somewhat less than in younger patients.

Guidelines for treatment with L-thyroxine are not well established for older patients who are found to have a raised level of TSH but who have normal serum thyroid hormone concentrations and few complaints. Such patients have subclinical hypothyroidism, and it is uncertain whether they suffer any significant disability from their minimal degree of hormone deficiency. Your doctor's decision whether or not to recommend L-thyroxine treatment has to be carefully weighed against potential complications of treatment, particularly as related to your heart.

An older patient is more likely to have undiagnosed coronary artery disease. If treatment begins with too large a dose of thyroid hormone, the patient's metabolic rate will rise too quickly. This will increase the work of the heart more rapidly than can be accommodated for by the narrowed coronary arteries. The result is chest pain, and heart damage can occur. The doctor will therefore initially prescribe a small daily dosage of L-thyroxine, no more than 0.025 mg, and raise the dosage at intervals of one month or more.

If you are hypothyroid and treated in this manner, you should not expect rapid improvement in your symptoms, because it will take three or four months before your dosage of L-thyroxine will be in the therapeutic range of 0.05 to 0.1

mg. Treatment with L-thyroxine is quite safe as long as your doctor adheres to these principles of therapy.

If you have known coronary heart disease with a normal T_4 and a slightly elevated TSH, you probably should not be treated with L-thyroxine. The risk of treatment might be disproportionately high in relation to your potential improvement. In such a case, you should see your doctor for measurement of serum thyroid hormones and TSH every six months. Should your serum thyroid hormone concentration begin to decrease, or should you develop symptoms of hypothyroidism, therapy with L-thyroxine could then be discussed with your cardiologist or primary care physician and then cautiously administered.

Hyperthyroidism

Hyperthyroidism is also more difficult to detect in the older patient because it affects older people with less-pronounced symptoms than younger patients.

Symptoms

Most younger hyperthyroid patients experience a rapid heartbeat with palpitations, feelings of warmth, discomfort in a warm environment, excessive perspiration, increased appetite, frequent bowel movements, weight loss, nervousness, and tremors (see chapter 6).

All of these symptoms are significantly muted in older patients. In these patients, hyperthyroidism may result only in rapid heartbeat, an arrhythmia of the heart (see chapter 6), or weight loss. This lack of full-fledged hyperthyroid symptoms, which is often called *apathetic hyperthyroidism*, may be caused by a decrease in the receptors for the adrenaline-like hormones that occurs during normal aging.

Because you won't have the classical symptoms and signs of hyperthyroidism, your doctor will need to consider hyperthyroidism as the underlying cause of unexplained loss of appetite and weight loss, muscle weakness, abnormal rhythms of the heart (especially atrial fibrillation), heart failure, and a worsening of chest pain due to angina pectoris. While each of these complaints clearly has many possible causes, hyperthyroidism must be on the list of possibilities. This is true even though you have none of the typical indications of the disease.

Diagnosis and Treatment

If your doctor suspects hyperthyroidism, measurement of your serum T_4 and TSH levels is sufficient to confirm the diagnosis. You should have a raised level of serum T_4, and your serum TSH should be less than 0.1 μU/ml. As in younger patients, the cause of your hyperthyroidism will be established by history, physical examination, and, if necessary, radioactive iodide uptake and scan (see chapters 5, 8, and 10). If you have thyroiditis, it will be self-limited, not requiring specific treatment. If you have Graves' disease or hyperthyroidism due to autonomous nodules, which is as common as Graves' disease in older patients, treatment with radioactive iodide or antithyroid drugs is appropriate (see chapters 8 and 9).

SUBCLINICAL HYPERTHYROIDISM

There is some disagreement among endocrinologists about the significance of a decreased concentration of serum TSH, less than 0.1 μU/ml, but without an increase in serum T_4 or T_3 concentration in elderly patients. These findings suggest subclinical hyperthyroidism (see chapters 8 and 10).

If you have blood levels consistent with subclinical hyperthyroidism and you are in good health, without any of the symptoms of hyperthyroidism that occur either in younger or older patients, you should probably not be given specific treatment but just observed every three to six months. You can always be treated if symptoms develop or if your serum thyroid hormone concentrations begin to rise—an indication of progressive worsening of your hyperthyroidism. Each case must be individualized. A second opinion might be worthwhile.

If you do have any of the symptoms of hyperthyroidism or if you also have heart disease, treatment of your subclinical hyperthyroidism will probably be beneficial to you because it may decrease the work load of your heart.

THE THYROID AND OBESITY

Many people who are overweight believe that their obesity is caused by an "underactive thyroid," and they may have actually received thyroid hormone treatment for weight reduction. The popular idea that hypothyroidism causes obesity originated long before accurate blood tests became available to measure thyroid hormones and TSH.

In the past, measurements of metabolic rate (see chapter 3) were carried out in many physicians' offices to diagnose thyroid function. The basal (resting) metabolic rate, or BMR, is raised in hyperthyroidism and decreased in hypothyroidism. However, many obese patients were not in a resting state when they arrived at their doctors' offices, and the tests were not always well administered. Many patients who went to their doctors complaining of obesity and fatigue had an inaccurate measurement of BMR and were placed on thyroid hormone treatment, which usually did not help them lose weight.

METABOLISM AND OBESITY

Modern measurements of thyroid hormones and TSH in the blood serum have led to a better understanding of the relationship of thyroid function and obesity. About 80 to 90 percent of hyperthyroid patients who have an increase in their metabolic rate lose weight despite an increase in food intake. This implies that their increased expenditure of energy due to increased BMR and physical activity is greater than their increase in energy intake in the form of food.

In contrast, hypothyroid patients seem to have only a moderate increase in weight, which results mainly from accumulation of fluid (see chapter 11). Although their metabolic rate is decreased, a reduction in food intake and in physical activity also occurs, usually resulting in normal energy balance, not in an accumulation of fat. Some hypothyroid patients give the appearance of obesity because of their fluid accumulation, which causes puffiness around their eyes, wrists, hands, and feet.

HYPOTHYROIDISM AND WEIGHT GAIN

If you are basically a lean person and you develop hypothyroidism, you may experience puffiness in your hands and feet and around your eyes, which will result in a weight gain of five to ten pounds. You should anticipate losing this extra weight once you are restored to the euthyroid state by thyroid hormone treatment (see chapter 13).

If you were obese before you developed hypothyroidism, you will gain only a moderate amount of weight because of the accumulation of fluid. With thyroid hormone treatment to restore you to the euthyroid state, you should lose the five to ten pounds of fluid but not your excess body fat. Many patients who are both obese and hypothyroid believe that their newly discovered hypothyroidism is the reason that they have been obese for many years, but this is rarely the case. For every 100 obese individuals, perhaps one or two have a significant degree of hypothyroidism and lose a significant amount of weight once they are treated with L-thyroxine.

EFFECTS OF L-THYROXINE

Your doctor will inform you to not expect lifelong obesity to melt away simply because you are taking L-thyroxine to treat your hypothyroidism. Obesity itself is a complex problem. If you have been obese for many years, you will have an increased number of fat cells and a propensity for storing more fat in your body than do lean individuals. These factors will strongly influence your obesity. Since neither of these biological factors is affected by your thyroid, you will not begin to lose large amounts of fat when you are treated with thyroid hormone.

Many patients who have not been informed of these distinctions will become disappointed with the result of L-thyroxine treatment because they have not had a large weight loss. Some patients may pressure their physicians to prescribe larger doses of L-thyroxine than are necessary, believing that a larger dose should produce more weight loss.

Inappropriate Thyroid Hormone Treatment

While it is true that an excessive dose of L-thyroxine produces hyperthyroidism, raises your energy expenditure, and results in weight loss, an overdose of L-thyroxine is not a safe way to lose weight and should be avoided. Excessive doses of thyroid hormone can result in all of the symptoms of hyperthyroidism, impair the function of your heart, cause abnormal heart rhythms, and lead to a loss of calcium from the bones.

If you are obese and believe you may have a "gland problem," you should go to your family physician or to an internist for a complete history and physical examination. Very few glandular disorders are associated with significant obesity, and those that are can readily be detected by your doctor by history, examination, and selected blood tests. If your serum T_4 and TSH blood levels are within the normal range, you should accept the fact that your thyroid function is normal, that your thyroid is not responsible in any way for your obesity, and that you will not benefit from thyroid hormone treatment. Your weight problem should then be treated by an appropriate decrease in your food intake and increase in your energy expenditure, usually by means of a progressive exercise program.

You should beware of the few doctors who prescribe L-thyroxine for obesity even though your serum T_4 and TSH are both normal. Such poorly informed or unscrupulous doctors believe that your obesity is caused by "hypometabolism without hypothyroidism," or that your body may not be producing sufficient amounts of T_4 from T_3 (see chapter 2). Therefore, the thinking goes, treatment with thyroid hormones—specifically L-triiodothyronine (*Cytomel*)—will reverse your obesity.

No medical evidence supporting these views has ever been reported. Therefore, if L-thyroxine or L-triiodothyronine treatment is recommended despite normal serum T_4 and TSH values, you should obtain a second opinion from an internist or endocrinologist before starting therapy. L-thyroxine treatment is a lifelong commitment and should be initiated only for medically valid reasons (see chapter 13).

Appendix

DIRECTORIES OF PHYSICIANS

Found in medical and many public libraries, these directories list information on virtually all physicians in the United States.

1.   American Medical Association Directory

The American Medical Association
Division of Survey and Data Resources
515 North State Street
Chicago, IL 60610

2.   Directory of Medical Specialists

Marquis Who's Who
Macmillan Directory Division
3002 Glenview Road
Wilmette, IL 60091

3. American Board of Medical Specialties Compendium of Certified Medical Specialists

The American Board of Medical Specialties
1 Rotary Center
Evanston, IL 60201

In addition, most state medical societies publish medical directories listing all physicians in the state. These directories also include information about their training and board certification.

PROFESSIONAL SOCIETIES

The Endocrine Society and the American Thyroid Association will help you find a physician who has the expertise to diagnose and manage your thyroid disease.

The *Endocrine Society* fosters research, training, and patient care for all endocrine diseases, including thyroid diseases.

Endocrine Society
9650 Rockville Pike
Bethesda, MD 20814-3998
301-571-1802

The society will provide you with the name of the director of the endocrinology training program that is nearest to you (usually a medical school or a major teaching hospital). You may then contact the training program director to obtain the name of a specific consultant in your area.

The American Thyroid Association is an organization that fosters research, training, and care of patients with thyroid diseases, specifically. If you contact the association, it will provide you with information about common thyroid diseases. It will also provide the names of several doctors in your area who have an interest and experience in treating patients with thyroid disorders.

Montefiore Medical Center
111 East 210th Street
Bronx, NY 10467
Physician referral tel. 1-800-542-6687

LAY ORGANIZATIONS

The Thyroid Foundation of America and The Thyroid Society for Education and Research are groups consisting of physicians who are expert in thyroid diseases and laypeople whose principal goals are patient education and support. If you contact these organizations, they will provide you with educational material concerning thyroid diseases and will also provide the names of physicians in your area who are qualified to treat your thyroid disorder.

Thyroid Foundation of America, Inc.
Ruth Sleeper Hall 350
40 Parkman Street
Boston, MA 02114
617-726-8500

The Thyroid Society for Education and Research
7515 South Main Street, Suite 545
Houston, TX 77030
1-800-THYROID (1-800-849-7643)

GLOSSARY

Adrenaline (epinephrine)—hormone that is secreted by the adrenal medulla (central portion of the adrenal gland) and certain nerve endings

Amino acids—building blocks for proteins

Angina pectoris—chest pain caused by inadequate blood flow to the heart muscle

Antibodies—proteins produced by special blood cells in response to specific antigens from either outside or inside the body (auto-antibodies)

Arrhythmia—abnormal heart rhythm

Autoimmunity—development of antibodies directed against one's own tissues

Binding proteins—proteins in serum that bind T_4 and T_3

BMR—basal metabolic rate

Bruit—noise related to increased blood flow through the thyroid; heard with a stethoscope

Calcitonin—hormone made by nonthyroid cells in the thyroid gland that helps prevent osteoporosis

Cataract—opacity in the lens of the eye

Colloid—protein-containing material surrounded by thyroid cells

Cornea—thin layer of cells that covers the pupil and iris of the eye

Cortisol—principal hormone secreted by the adrenal cortex

Cretinism—congenital hypothyroidism

Cricoid cartilage—cartilage just below the thyroid cartilage

CT (CAT)—computerized axial tomography; an X-ray procedure that provides images of the internal organs of the body

Dexamethasone—synthetic glucocorticoid

Diplopia—double vision; two objects will be seen when there is actually one

Dysphagia—difficulty in swallowing food or liquids

Endocrine gland—ductless gland that produces hormones that enter the bloodstream and act at distant sites in the body

Esophagus—muscular tube that carries food from mouth to stomach

Estrogen—female sex hormone

Euthyroid—normal thyroid state

Exophthalmometer—device to measure how far each eye is protruding

Exophthalmopathy—eye disorder that occurs in Graves' disease

Exophthalmos—protruding eyes

Follicle-stimulating hormone (FSH)—pituitary hormone that regulates egg development in the ovary or sperm development in the testes

Gene—portion of DNA containing the chemical code that dictates the formation of a specific messenger RNA

Glucocorticoid—hormone made in the adrenal cortex that stimulates sugar formation and maintains blood vessel tone

Goiter—enlarged thyroid

Graves' disease—autoimmune thyroid disease that causes hyperthyroidism and orbitopathy

Hashimoto's thyroiditis—autoimmune thyroid disease that causes hypothyroidism

Hormones—chemical messengers produced by endocrine glands

Hyperthyroidism—overactive thyroid

Hypoparathyroidism—decreased function of the parathyroid glands

Hypothalamus—area in base of brain containing cells that produce hormones to stimulate or inhibit release of pituitary hormones

Hypothyroidism—underactive thyroid

Larynx—voice box

Luteinizing hormone (LH)—pituitary hormone that regulates hormone production in the ovary or testosterone secretion in the testes

Messenger RNA—substance containing the chemical code of a specific gene; it dictates the sequence of amino acids in a specific protein

Methimazole—antithyroid drug

GLOSSARY

MRI—magnetic resonance imaging, a procedure that enables visualization of soft tissues without the use of X rays

Myocardial infarction—heart attack

Myxedema—severe form of hypothyroidism

Negative feedback—ability of T_4 and T_3 to inhibit the secretion of TSH

Optic nerve—nerve in back of eye that transmits visual signals to the brain

Orbit—bony socket of the skull that contains the eyeball, eye muscles, blood vessels, and nerves

Orbitopathy—disorder of eye muscles and contents of the orbit that occurs in Graves' disease

Palpitation—feeling of rapid heartbeat, forceful heartbeat, or irregular heartbeat

Parathyroid glands—four small glands located behind the thyroid (two on each side) that produce parathyroid hormone

Parathyroid hormone—regulates the blood calcium level by acting on bone and kidney

Paroxysmal atrial fibrillation—sudden onset of rapid and irregular heart rhythm

Pituitary—"master gland"—glandular tissue connected at the base of the brain by a stalk; secretes growth hormone, prolactin, and hormones that regulate the thyroid, adrenals, ovaries, and testicles

Plasma—yellowish fluid that remains in unclotted blood after all blood cells have been removed

Prolactin—pituitary hormone that regulates milk production by the breast

Proptosis—bulging eyes

Propylthiouracil (PTU)—antithyroid drug

Receptor—cell protein that binds T_4 or T_3 and regulates specific genes

Secretion—process by which hormones enter the bloodstream

Serum—yellowish fluid that remains after blood has clotted

Syndrome—group of symptoms and signs common to a patient with a specific disorder

T_3—abbreviation for triiodothyronine

T_4—abbreviation for thyroxine

Tapazole—antithyroid drug (see methimazole)

Testosterone—male sex hormone

Thyroglobulin—unique thyroid protein

Thyroid cartilage—contains the voice box (larynx)

Thyroidectomy—surgical removal of the thyroid

Thyroid gland—endocrine gland located in the front part of the neck that produces thyroid hormones

Thyroid nodule—lump in the thyroid gland

Thyroid peroxidase—thyroid protein (enzyme) that facilitates introduction of iodine into another thyroid protein, thyroglobulin

Thyroid-stimulating antibody (TSAb)—binds to TSH receptor and produces hyperthyroidism in Graves' disease

Thyrotrophin-releasing hormone (TRH)—hormone from the hypothalamus that causes secretion of TSH from the pituitary

Thyroxine (T_4)—thyroid hormone that contains four iodine atoms

Trachea—breathing tube, or windpipe

Triiodothyronine (T_3)—thyroid hormone that contains three iodine atoms

TSAb—thyroid-stimulating antibody

TSH—thyroid-stimulating hormone made in pituitary gland

TSH receptor—protein on surface of thyroid cells that binds TSH and transmits its chemical message to the cell

Ultrasound examination, or sonogram of thyroid—image of the thyroid gland produced with ultrasonic (high-frequency sound) waves

INDEX

in thyroiditis, 132, 137–40
treatment of, 122–31
weight gain and, 196–97

Imaging tests, 28, 50–51
Inderal, 78
Infertility, 106, 173
Inflammation of thyroid. *See*
  Thyroiditis
Iodide, 6–7
  deficiency of, 115, 142
  excess intake of, 115–17, 146
  solutions, 76–77, 81
Isthmus, 5–6

Larynx, 5, 80
Lid lag, 49
Light, sensitivity to, 84
Lithium, 117–18
Lobectomy, 161
L-thyroxine, 123–31, 137, 139,
  147–48, 150, 157–58, 178
  for children, 185
  for elderly, 191
  obesity and, 197–98
  during pregnancy, 174, 175
Lugol's solution, 76
Lymph nodes, enlarged, 162,
  163, 170
Lymphocytes, 107
Lymphocytic thyroiditis, 138–40

Magnetic resonance imaging
  (MRI), 28, 50–51, 144
Medical history, 21–22
Medications. *See* Drugs
Medullary cancer, 153, 169–70
Menstrual disorders, 39
  in hypothyroidism, 106, 172
Messenger RNA, 12, 13

Metabolism, 15
  heart changes and, 16
  measurement of, 195
  obesity and, 196
Metastases, 165, 169
Methimazole, 55, 57–62, 64,
  175, 177, 178
Miscarriage, 39, 173, 177
Muscle changes, 14
  in hyperthyroidism, 38–39
  in hypothyroidism, 105
Myocardial infarction, 17
Myxedema, 3–4, 101

Nail changes, 14
  in hyperthyroidism, 35
  in hypothyroidism, 101
Necklace incision, 162
Neck pain, 133–34
  in cancer, 151
Negative-feedback regulation of
  TSH, 11
Neurological disorders, 36–37
  in hypothyroidism, 104–5
Newborn, hyperthyroidism and,
  177–78
Nodules, 19, 22, 90–97, 142,
  143, 145, 149–58
  assessment of, 28
  diagnosis of, 91–93
  differential diagnosis of cancer
    and, 149–57
  evaluation of, 150
  radioactive iodide treatment
    for, 96–97
  surgery for, 95–96, 113
  timing of treatment of, 94–95
Nuclear Regulatory Commission,
  166
Nursing mothers, 178